The Modern Medical Office:
A Reference Manual

Doris Humphrey, Ph.D.
Chairperson
Department of Office Administration
Raymond Walters Community College
University of Cincinnati
Cincinnati, Ohio

Kathie Sigler, Ed.D.
Dean for Administration
Miami-Dade Community College
Miami, Florida

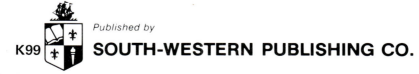

Published by
SOUTH-WESTERN PUBLISHING CO.

CINCINNATI   WEST CHICAGO, IL   DALLAS   PELHAM MANOR, NY   LIVERMORE, CA

Copyright © 1986
by South-Western Publishing Co.
Cincinnati, Ohio

All Rights Reserved

The text of this publication, or any part thereof, may not be reproduced or transmitted in any form or by any means, electronic or mechanical, including photocopying, recording, storage in an information retrieval system, or otherwise, without the prior written permission of the publisher.

ISBN: 0-538-11990-X

Library of Congress Catalog
Card Number: 85-50551

3 4 5 Ki 0 9 8 7

Printed in the United States of America

Preface

Medical office personnel face special challenges as they make the transition from traditional to contemporary office procedures. While some tasks have remained the same, others have been affected by tremendous advances in office technology. For example, good human relations skills have not changed; therefore, traditional methods of greeting and working with patients are still very valuable. However, accounting, billing, creating and storing correspondence, and other office tasks have undergone great change through the use of computers.

This reference manual attempts to prepare individuals to work in either a traditional medical office or a contemporary medical office. You will find a broad spectrum of topics—from alphabetic and numeric filing to computerized account management. You'll find diverse chapters such as Medical Ethics and Medical Law, Punctuation, and Travel Arrangements. This manual is a handy guide no matter how limited or extensive your medical office background.

Several institutions, physicians, and individuals contributed to the material in this book. In particular, we would like to thank the reviewers, Linda Ballhaus, R.N., Southern Ohio College, Cincinnati, Ohio and Mary M. Haugen, CMA-AC, Indiana Vocational Technical College, Ft. Wayne, Indiana. We would also like to thank Bethesda North Hospital, Cincinnati, Ohio; Jackson Memorial Hospital, Miami, Florida; William M. Humphrey, M.D.; Kenneth D. Stringer, D.O.; John Tholking, M.D.; Marlene Evans, Medical Office Manager; Donna McSpadden, Medical Office Manager; and Zoila de Zayas, Miami-Dade Community College.

Doris Humphrey
Kathie Sigler

Contents

THE MODERN MEDICAL OFFICE
1. Overview 1
2. Medical Ethics and Medical Law 18

MEDICAL COMMUNICATIONS
3. Interpersonal Skills 35
4. Telephone Communication 47
5. Medical Forms and Medical Reports 60
6. Medical Correspondence 79

MEDICAL OFFICE PROCEDURES
7. Medical Office Files 105
8. Scheduling 131
9. Travel Arrangements 142

INSURANCE AND ACCOUNTING PROCEDURES
10. Health Insurance 148
11. Accounting Procedures in the Medical Office 166
12. Medical Billing and Collections 177

MEDICAL OFFICE TECHNOLOGY
13. Word Processing in the Medical Office 190
14. The Computer in the Medical Office 202

LANGUAGE USAGE

    15   Parts of Speech   218

    16   Eliminating Bias in Writing   233

    17   Punctuation   237

    18   Capitalization   252

    19   Hyphenation   260

APPENDIX   264

    Common Medical Terminology

    Abridged List of Medical Abbreviations, Symbols, and Terms

    Professional Organizations and Information

INDEX   281

1

Overview

TYPES OF MEDICAL FACILITIES

Medical offices vary in size and physicians' specialities, but the office duties performed in each are very similar. Medical office workers handle a variety of tasks, including patient scheduling, typing, general accounting, answering the telephone, and greeting patients. Most medical offices employ only a small number of office workers; but taken as a whole, medical offices provide many employment opportunities. Employment opportunities exist in the following types of medical facilities.

1.1 Traditional Medical Offices

Traditional medical offices center around the practices of one to three doctors. These small offices may consist of doctors practicing the same or different medical specialities. Employees in small medical offices handle a variety of duties each day.

1.2 Medical Centers

Many doctors work together in *medical centers*. These centers are sometimes based on one speciality, such as surgery, with member physicians further specializing in specific types of surgery. Other medical centers are comprised of physicians with widely varied specialities, thus providing a patient with a full complement of medical services within one office. Several office workers in a medical center might share office responsibilities, or specific tasks might be assigned to each office worker.

1.3 Hospitals

Hospitals are large-scale medical office employers. In hospitals, medical office workers are generally assigned to specific departments or divisions with very specialized tasks. One employee might assist with the complex task of organizing the surgical schedule, while another might work solely in the hospital accounting department.

1.4 Research Centers

Research centers are devoted to the in-depth study of medical problems. They are generally connected to a university or a hospital, and they provide many employment opportunities for medical office workers. As in the case of hospitals, jobs in these centers are likely to be specialized according to the department or division assignment.

1.5 Other Medical Office Employers

Medical office workers will also find positions in university medical schools, pharmaceutical companies, and in businesses which manufacture medical supplies and equipment.

1.6 Speciality Areas of Physicians

The following are the most common types of medical practices:

- *Ear, Nose, and Throat (ENT)*—treatment of diseases related to the ears, nose, and throat.

- *General Practice or Family Practice*—treatment of the entire family for the prevention and cure of common illnesses.

- *Internal Medicine*—treatment of nonsurgical conditions such as heart disease.

- *Neurology*—treatment of diseases of the brain, spinal cord, and the rest of the nervous system.

- *Obstetrics/Gynecology (OB/GYN)*—treatment of pregnancies and diseases of the female reproductive system.

- *Ophthalmology*—treatment of diseases of the eyes.

- *Orthopedics*—treatment of diseases of the bones.

- *Pediatrics*—treatment of infants and children.

- *Surgery*—treatment of diseases and injuries through the performance of operations. Many surgeons specialize in specific areas of surgery.

- *Urology*—treatment of diseases of the urinary system. *Nephrology* is a speciality where physicians concentrate on medical conditions related to the kidneys, such as dialysis.

FINDING EMPLOYMENT IN THE MEDICAL FIELD

To successfully find employment in the medical field, one of the first things you need to know is what employers are looking for. The following skills are most requested by medical employers today:

1. **Basic Academic Skills.** These skills involve the ability to read, write, compute, and think logically. Today these skills are a problem for many office workers. Good skills in grammar and spelling are essential to the production of error-free office correspondence.

2. **Secretarial Skills.** These skills involve the ability to type quickly and accurately, to transcribe accurately from machine dictation, to arrange typed material attractively on a page, to file and retrieve materials, and to use good telephone etiquette.

3. **Human Relations.** These skills involve the ability to deal with people in a pleasant, friendly manner. The medical office employee needs to be able to get along with supervisors, fellow workers, and patients. Often the first contact a patient has with the medical office is with the office personnel. It is important that these interactions be positive. Employers are looking for medical office workers who can maintain a cheerful attitude, even in times of stress.

4. **Medical Knowledge, Experience, and Skills.** You may be surprised to learn that these skills, while desirable, are ranked as the least important for the medical office employee to possess. If you have the skills mentioned in Items 1-3 above, the medical office will be willing to teach you the specific medical knowledge you need. At the same time, if you are strong in Items 1-3, additional medical knowledge will make you the strongest possible candidate for a job opening. The most sought-after qualities in this category are knowledge of medical terminology and actual work experience in the medical field.

1.7 Where to Look for Employment Possibilities

Job opportunities should be open to all regardless of sex, race, ethnic heritage, religion, creed, age, or physical disability.

Posted or Advertised Positions. Look through job openings already advertised or posted. There are many places where you can find such notices of medical office positions. Some are listed below.

- The classified section of a newspaper
- Public or private employment agencies (WARNING: If you use an employment agency, make sure you know who pays the agency fee, if

there is one. It is not wise to pay a fee to an agency yourself unless you first obtain a job through their efforts. Many times the employer pays the employment agency fee.)

- School bulletin boards or placement offices
- Magazines, professional medical journals, periodicals
- Bulletin boards in medical offices, research centers, medical centers, hospitals, pharmaceutical companies, and medical equipment and supply manufacturers

Job Vacancies Not Yet Advertised.   There are several ways you can find out about job openings not yet advertised.

- Talk with family or friends. They may know of upcoming employment opportunities in the medical field.
- Visit personnel offices of medical employers. Since personnel offices are responsible for posting and advertising all employment openings, a visit will often provide valuable information on upcoming openings.
- Look for new or expanding medical facilities. The local newspaper often contains information regarding the opening of new medical offices, medically related businesses, or medical schools within a university. The opening or expansion of any of these would require additional personnel.

1.8   Job Inquiry Letter

Once you know of job possibilities, making a personal visit or writing a *job inquiry letter* (see Figure 1-1) is your next step. You may wish to send the inquiry letter on cream-colored, grey, or beige paper. Using colored paper for your cover letter, envelope, and résumé can make your inquiry stand out from the rest. The final package sent to the employer should contain no strikeovers; all corrections should be neatly made and not obvious to the reader.

Review the Yellow Pages of the telephone directory to find potential medical employers. Once you have a list of possibilities, send a job inquiry letter (Figure 1-1) along with your résumé to the medical employer.

1.9   Application Forms

When you write, call, or visit a medical employer during an employment search, you will usually be asked to fill out an *application form*. The application form requests similar information to that given in your résumé. You should have your résumé available when complet-

Figure 1-1 Job Inquiry Letter

9090 S.W. 85 Avenue
Miami, FL 33156-4563
June 1, 19--

Ms. Annie Betancourt
Personnel Manager
Jackson Memorial Hospital
1611 N.W. 12th Avenue
Miami, FL 33136-5050

Dear Ms. Betancourt:

The article in the May 20, 19-- issue of <u>The Miami Herald</u> about the upcoming expansion of the Pediatric Care Unit at Jackson Memorial Hospital was very interesting to me. One of my neighbor's children received excellent care from the doctors and nurses in the Pediatric Care Unit following a recent automobile accident. I am happy to see this expansion, since it will ensure the same quality treatment for many other children.

Since this new expansion will require additional personnel, could the Pediatric Care Unit use a secretary who:

1. will work with little supervision, and will take the initiative in completing complex tasks?

2. will be dependable and punctual?

3. will work well with the public?

If so, I am the medical secretary for you!

The Pediatric Care Unit needs medical secretaries who recognize the importance of accurate medical records and careful treatment of patients. These areas were stressed in my medical transcription training at Miami-Dade Community College.

If you decide to add me to your medical team, Jackson Memorial Hospital would be assured of a dedicated medical transcriptionist who sincerely cares for children.

In your hiring for the expanded Pediatric Care Unit, please give serious consideration to the enclosed resume. To arrange an interview, call me at 555-5122. I look forward to hearing from you soon.

Sincerely,

Zoila de Zayas

Zoila de Zayas

Enclosure

ing your application so that all dates and other information are accurate.

Since your application form, application letter, and résumé will be the three written items considered before an interview is granted, it is important that all three represent you well. If you have the opportunity, ask to complete the application form at home so that you can neatly type the information requested. If you are requested to complete the form in the employer's office, do so neatly and in ink (see Figure 1-2).

Read through the entire form before you fill it out, and note all of the questions asked. You will avoid putting answers in the wrong blanks by reviewing the form first. Follow directions carefully, watching for instructions such as "last name first." Fill the form out completely. Answer all questions fully and accurately. If any question cannot be answered (for example, information requested on military service if you have not been in the military), put *NA* on the blank line to show that the question is not applicable to you, and to show that you did not miss answering the question. All information provided on the application form and résumé should agree exactly. If asked for a desired salary, provide a salary range rather than a specific amount. This will leave the subject open for discussion during the interview.

When you have completed the application form, review it carefully to make certain you have filled out each line with the information requested. Then attach a copy of your résumé to the completed application form before submitting both to the employer.

1.10 Employment Tests

Employment tests are given by medical employers to obtain additional information about prospective employees. The results of these tests are considered in the selection of medical employees, but sometimes tests can be retaken to improve your score. Employment tests may cover typing, shorthand, medical terminology, general intelligence, personality, or math. If you have received any certificates from school indicating your proficiency in any of these areas, take these certificates with you to the employment office. Medical offices will sometimes accept such credentials and excuse you from the employment test covering the certified skills. Remember the following things if you are asked to take an employment test:

- Relax as much as possible.
- Read all instructions carefully. If you are being given a timed test, request time to read instructions before the timed portion begins. Ask questions if you do not understand any directions.

Chapter 1—Overview

Figure 1-2 Application Form

Jackson Memorial Hospital
the health team that cares.
Application for Employment

INSTRUCTIONS: This application must be filled out personally. Use black or blue ink. False or misleading statements are cause for rejection. All statements are subject to investigation. Answer all questions accurately and completely. PLEASE PRINT CLEARLY.

Position(s) applied for: **MEDICAL SECRETARY** / **MEDICAL TRANSCRIBER**

LAST NAME: (Print in Full)	First Name	Middle/Maiden Name	Social Security Number
de ZAYAS	ZOILA	ESTHER	263-74-3859

Present Address Street	Residence Telephone
9090 S.W. 85 AVENUE	(305) 555-5122

City	State	Zip Code	Other phone numbers where you may be contacted
MIAMI	FL	33156-4563	MOTHER 555-7482

Are you a citizen of the U.S.? Yes ☒ No ☐ If no, do you have a legal right to remain and work in the United States? Yes ☐ No ☐

EDUCATION TRAINING

Foreign Language Proficiency - Print the word "Good," "Fair," or "Poor" in the boxes titled Read, Write, Speak which best describes your ability to use this language.

Place "X" in column indicating highest grade completed

Language	Read	Write	Speak
SPANISH	GOOD	GOOD	GOOD

5	6	7	8	9	10	11	12	GED	COLLEGE
									A.S. X

	Name and Location	Dates From To	Graduated?	Major & Minor Subjects	Degree	Activities or Honors
High School	CORAL GABLES HIGH SCHOOL CORAL GABLES, FL.	19- 19-	YES	COLLEGE PREP/ BUSINESS EDUCATION	DIPLO MA	NAT'L HONOR SOCIETY ST. COUNCIL VICE-PRESIDENT
College	MITCHELL WOLFSON NEW WORLD CENTER CAMPUS MIAMI-DADE COMM. COLLEGE MIAMI, FL.	19- 19-	YES	MEDICAL TRANSCRIPTION MAJOR	A.S.	ASST. EDITOR, METROPOLIS, PRESIDENT, PI THETA KAPPA
Other	NA					

Occupational or professional license(s)
If you have one: Type **CERTIFICATE FROM M-DCC**   Number **NONE**
Date obtained **MARCH 19,** _____ Renewal Date **NA**
If one is pending: Type **NA**   Date to be received **NA**
OTHER SKILLS: Typing **60** wpm   Shorthand/Speedwriting **100** wpm
Other: **WORD PROCESSING EQUIPMENT, KNOWLEDGE OF MEDICAL TERMINOLOGY, MED. TRANSCRIPT.**

Have you ever been a member of the Armed Services?	☐ Yes ☒ No	Type of discharge: ☐ Honorable ☐ Other (Explain)	Date of Discharge
Dates, From **NA** To _____		**NA**	Month Day Year **NA**

8 The Modern Medical Office

Figure 1-2 (continued)

V. Health Record

Do you have any reason that precludes you from performing any part of the job for which you are being considered? _____
NONE, EXCELLENT HEALTH

Since your 16th birthday, have you ever been ☐ Yes   If "Yes," state the court, nature of offense, disposition of case
convicted of a felonious offense?   ☒ No   and date. NA

Prior to employment, your fingerprints will be taken for routine check by the F.B.I. and other agencies.

Employment Record

Have you been previously employed by   If "Yes," state department and dates
Jackson Memorial Hospital? Yes ☐ No ☒   NA

List in order, starting with present or last employer.

Dates Month Year	Company		Telephone
	BAPTIST HOSPITAL		555-8076
	Street 8500 S.W. 89 STREET	City MIAMI	State FL Zip 33156-7753
From: APRIL 19—	Job Title VOLUNTEER	Department VOLUNTEER SERVICES	Supervisor DR. CASTELL BRYANT
	Major Duties TYPING, FILING, DELIVERY, CANDY/MAGAZINE CART, WORD PROCESSING		
To: PRESENT	Starting Salary $ NA Per NA	Final Salary $ NA Per NA	Reason for leaving STILL A VOLUNTEER
	Company CHICKEN SHACK		Telephone 555-1191
	Street 11905 S.W. 88 STREET	City MIAMI	State FL Zip 33176-7746
From: AUGUST 19—	Job Title COOK	Department KITCHEN	Supervisor MR. LOUIS MONZON
	Major Duties FOOD PREPARATION		
To: PRESENT	Starting Salary $3.35 Per HOUR	Final Salary $3.70 Per HOUR	Reason for leaving STILL WORKING
	Company NA		Telephone
	Street	City	State Zip
From:	Job Title	Department	Supervisor
	Major Duties		
To:	Starting Salary $ Per	Final Salary $ Per	Reason for leaving
	Company NA		Telephone
	Street	City	State Zip
From:	Job Title	Department	Supervisor
	Major Duties		
To:	Starting Salary $ Per	Final Salary $ Per	Reason for leaving
	Company NA		Telephone
	Street	City	State Zip
From:	Job Title	Department	Supervisor
	Major Duties		
To:	Starting Salary $ Per	Final Salary $ Per	Reason for leaving

CERTIFICATION: I hereby certify that all statements made on this form are true to the best of my knowledge. I fully realize that should an investigation disclose any misrepresentation, I will be subject to immediate dismissal.

Date: 6/29/—   Signature: Y. deGayas

We are an Equal Opportunity Employer and participate in Affirmative Action Programs. Our application forms are designed to obtain an applicant's skills, knowledge and abilities based on specific job requirements. Questions are designed to elicit enough data for us to determine an applicant's abilities to successfully perform the job for which she/he is applying.

- Use your time wisely. Divide your allotted time to make sure you have time for each section of the test. Don't waste time on one particular question. Skip the troublesome questions and come back to them later, if you have time.

- Look for answers to harder questions in other parts of the test. You will be surprised how many hints you may find.

- Write clearly and neatly so your answers can be read.

In addition to a test of your medical office skills, many medical employers will require a physical examination. This is usually for insurance purposes and to make sure you do not have any illness or disease that would interfere with your performance on the job or be transmitted to patients or co-workers

1.11 The Résumé

Type your *résumé* neatly since it is a written picture of you—your experience, your skills, and your abilities (See Figure 1-3). It is one of the best tools you have to convince an employer to grant you a personal interview. The résumé is sometimes referred to as the personal data sheet or curriculum vitae.

If you type your cover letter on light-colored stationery, you should type your résumé to match. Putting the cover letter and résumé on colored paper can make your application stand out from the rest. Your résumé will consist of the following general sections:

1. **Personal Information.** Include your name, address, and telephone number. Review this information for accuracy. Height, weight, marital status, number of children, birth date, social security number, health, and birthplace are sometimes included in this section, but recent laws preventing discrimination in hiring have made these items optional.

2. **Education.** Include the degrees you have earned, listing the most recent first. Show the dates of your attendance at each school. Indicate the school, college, or university where your degree was awarded; the location of your school (city/state); your major (minor optional); and the month and year your degree was awarded.

3. **Work Experience.** Beginning with your most recent job, list your job titles, names of the companies and their locations (city/state), and dates of employment. If you do not have much paid work experience, list volunteer work in this category and clearly indicate that you were a volunteer worker. Optional items in this category include the name and title of your direct supervisor and job duties and responsibilities.

4. **Other Categories.** While the categories above are always included on a résumé, the following categories are optional, allowing you to choose

Figure 1-3 A Résumé

Zoila de Zayas
9090 S.W. 85 Avenue
Miami, FL 33156-4563
(305) 555-5122

EDUCATION

September, 19-- to
August, 19--

Mitchell Wolfson New World
  Center Campus
Miami-Dade Community College
Miami, Florida
Medical Transcription
Degree: A.S., August, 19--

September, 19-- to
June, 19--

Coral Gables High School
Coral Gables, Florida
College Prep/Business Education
Diploma: June, 19--

WORK EXPERIENCE

August, 19-- to Present

Cook
Chicken Shack, Miami, Florida
Mr. Louis Monzon, Manager
This position has helped me pay
  for my college education.

April, 19-- to Present

Volunteer
Baptist Hospital, Miami, Florida
Dr. Castell Bryant, Volunteer
  Coordinator
Type, file, deliver candy and
  magazines, and use word pro-
  cessing equipment.

SPECIAL SKILLS

Occupational Skills:

Typing 60 wpm
Shorthand 100 wpm
Word Processing Equipment
Medical Terminology
Medical Dictation/
  Transcription

COLLEGE ACTIVITIES

Assistant Editor, School Newspaper; President (19--), Pi
  Theta Kappa Honorary Society

Zoila de Zayas
Page 2

HONORS AND AWARDS

19--   Silver Knight Award in Business,
                            The Miami Herald

REFERENCES (WITH PERMISSION)

Castell Bryant, M.D.   Mr. Louis Monzon, Manager
Volunteer Coordinator   Chicken Shack
Baptist Hospital   11905 S.W. 88 Street
8900 S.W. 89 Street   Miami, FL 33176-7746
Miami, FL 33176-7753   (305) 555-1191
(305) 555-8076

         Ms. Lynn Forrester
         Department Chairperson
         Office Technology Department
         Mitchell Wolfson New World Center Campus
         Miami-Dade Community College
         300 N.E. 2nd Avenue
         Miami, FL 33132-7705
         (305) 555-6800

from among them to present your "written picture" in the best possible way:

- **a. Special Skills.** Information in this category includes job-related courses you have taken or skills you have attained.

- **b. High School or College Activities.** Include the names of organizations or clubs of which you were a member, the offices you held, and the years you were a member. You might also mention any special activities that you organized.

- **c. Special Honors or Awards.** Include any special honors or awards you have received.

- **d. Service to the Community.** Include any community activities, professional memberships, etc.

- **e. Military Service.** Include the branch of service, rank, dates of service, military occupation or specialty, and any awards or honors.

- **f. Hobbies or Special Interests.**

- **g. References.** Be sure to get the consent of those whom you list as references. You should be certain that each one will know how to stress your particular skills. Indicate name, position, place of employment, business address, and phone number for each reference.

While each résumé contains similar categories, you may want to tailor your résumé to the position for which you are applying. For example, a position in a hospital accounting office would call for math, bookkeeping, and electronic calculator skills. A position at the reception desk would call for human relations skills and good telephone techniques. Put yourself in the position of the medical employer reading your résumé. Make certain you have answered all the questions this prospective employer might have.

While your résumé should be brief and concise, it will get longer as you gain work experience. When you need to add a second or third page, use the following heading:

```
Your Name
Page 2
```

1.12 Application Letter

The *application letter* introduces the résumé to the prospective medical employer. It points out your special skills and abilities and suggests that you be invited for a personal interview. In Figure 1-1, a job inquiry letter is shown. This type of letter is written to determine if there are any openings that fit your skills.

Figure 1-4 shows an ad for a vacant position. In response to such an ad, you might write an application letter such as that shown in Figure 1-5.

Figure 1-4 Job Opening Ad

Medical Transcriptionist
LET'S BUILD A FUTURE TOGETHER!
Knowledge of Medical terminology. 60+ wpm. Top pay. Community Health of Dade County. 555-9277

This sort of letter is aimed at a specific opening. The application letter must get the reader's attention, so find creative ways to distinguish yourself from other applicants. Read the first paragraphs of the letters shown in Figures 1-1 and 1-5 for attention-getting ideas

Highlight your qualifications and special skills to show how you could be the best candidate for the position. Elaborate on specific items in your résumé.

Ask for immediate action in the final paragraph of your application letter. Your request should be appropriate to the specific position for which you are applying. You might suggest a time when you can be reached or propose a day for an interview.

1.13   The Interview

The very best chance you have to convince a medical employer to hire you is the personal interview. During the interview you can have a detailed discussion of how your skills can assist a medical employer. At the same time, the interviewer will have a chance to evaluate your personality, attitudes, appearance, enthusiasm, and ability to communicate.

You should recognize that the interview is also an opportunity to evaluate the open position. You need to make certain that this medical office is one in which you would be happy.

Prepare First.   Before you go to the interview, learn all you can about the medical employer. Ask your teachers and friends about the skills normally required for the open position and make sure your skills are adequate. Find out what the salaries are for similar positions in your area so you will know what to expect, or what to answer if you are asked about salary. Be aware of fringe benefits provided by similar medical employers and decide which benefits are most important to you. Ask family and friends for possible interview questions so you

Figure 1-5 Application Letter

                                        9090 S.W. 85 Avenue
                                        Miami, FL 33156-4563
                                        June 1, 19--

Marcia Stringer, D.O.
Community Health of Dade County
10300 S.W. 216 Street
Miami, FL 33176-8560

Dear Dr. Stringer:

The future looks bright since your classified ad for a medical transcriptionist appeared in the May 27 issue of <u>The Miami Herald</u>. Your ad suggests, "Let's build a future together." Since I am beginning my career as a medical transcriber, I would be happy to help build your medical practice, too.

As you will note from my enclosed resume, <u>The Miami Herald</u> selected me as a candidate for future success by awarding me the coveted "Silver Knight" award in business during my senior year in high school. While paid working experience in a medical environment has not yet been possible, I have worked for several years as a volunteer at Baptist Hospital in South Dade. Some of this volunteer work has consisted of transcribing medical dictation. In addition, my courses at Miami-Dade Community College provided me with much practice in medical transcription; I received "A" grades in both Medical Terminology and Medical Transcription.

The future success of your medical office depends on dedicated, competent assistance. You can count on me. Please call me soon at 555-5122 for a personal interview.

                                        Sincerely,

                                        Zoila de Zayas

                                        Zoila de Zayas

Enclosure

can begin to think of good answers. Think of questions you may want to ask the interviewer and write them down to take with you. Arrange these questions in order of priority, in case you do not have time to ask them all.

Since this is the first opportunity the medical employer will have to judge your appearance, make sure you look your best. Decide in advance what to wear. Dress in your best business attire, and be sure your clothes are clean and wrinkle-free. Most important—remember to wear a smile!

Going to the Interview. Allow yourself plenty of time to dress and get to the interview. If you are not sure of the location, call for directions before leaving home.

During the Interview. Try to appear relaxed. While all candidates will be somewhat nervous during an interview, try not to show your uneasiness by squirming in your chair or tapping your fingers. An interview usually lasts about a half hour.

The interviewer will take charge of the interview with the first question. Listen to all questions carefully and ask for clarification if you are confused. Answer all questions honestly and briefly, but provide more than yes or no answers. Look the interviewer in the eye while speaking and smile often.

Remember that you are there to sell yourself. Think of all your skills and interests and discuss them in relation to the requirements for the position. Save your questions about the position and the employer until the end of the interview. While salary and benefits are important concerns, you should not focus all your questions on salary, vacations, and bonuses.

Avoid any criticism of past employers, teachers, or yourself. Keep the interview positive and forward-looking. Watch for indications from the interviewer that the interview is nearing an end. If you are interested in working for this medical office, close the interview by expressing your interest:

> Dr. Stringer, you've been very kind to take time from your busy schedule to talk to me. The information you have provided about your open position has been helpful. You can count on my dedication if I am given the opportunity to work with you.

1.14 Check Back

Write a brief thank-you letter to the interviewer a few days after the interview to help the interviewer remember you and your qualifications. The interviewer should be thanked for the time and attention. You should repeat your interest in the position. (See Figure 1-6.)

Figure 1-6 Thank-you Letter

9090 S.W. 85 Avenue
Miami, FL 33156-4563
June 15, 19--

Marcia Stringer, D.O.
Community Health of Dade County
10300 S.W. 216 Street
Miami, FL 33176-8560

Dear Dr. Stringer:

Thank you very much for taking the time from your busy schedule to meet with me last Wednesday. Your description of the job was quite comprehensive and very informative.

I am interested in working in an office such as you described. If you decide to give me the opportunity, I will strive to be accurate and dependable.

Sincerely,

Zoila de Zayas

Zoila de Zayas

1.15 Automated Office

When you begin a new job in a medical office, there may be many things you do not know or understand. Take the time to ask questions and to be sure you understand instructions. Admit mistakes readily. Approach your employer with any errors you discover and discuss frankly how to solve the problem. Assure your employer that you will take steps to avoid the problem in the future.

You will also find that office technology has significantly affected the job of the medical office employee. Word processing equipment allows for the easy revision and reorganization of typed material; it checks spelling and performs some simple computations. Future word processing equipment will do even more to ease the task of medical office workers.

Word processing and data processing are moving closer and closer together. Microcomputers function as both word processors and minicomputers with special software programs. This trend will continue.

New telephone technology will also change the medical office. There are now telephones that function as microcomputers and allow easy transmission of data via telephone lines. These same telephones will allow access to a mainframe computer so that information can be withdrawn from the memory of the computer and added to the text of a letter or report.

This technology is changing so rapidly that we all must continue to learn about how these machines can make the medical office more efficient, allowing more time for working personally with patients and staff. Later sections of this manual will cover the changing office environment in more detail.

1.16 How to Advance

While your first years on the job will be spent learning and perfecting your job skills, you should also begin thinking of goals for the future. Sometimes you can find better positions to aim for within your own organization. In other cases, career advancement requires changing medical employers. It is important to constantly keep your goals in mind.

Good advice for job advancement is to dress and act for a position you aspire to, rather than for the position you now have.

Continue Learning. If you are to advance within the medical profession, you must continue to improve and expand your knowledge. Most physicians firmly believe in continuing education for their employees because of their own continuing education requirements.

The medical office worker should show a willingness to learn, even on weekends and after office hours. If you learn of any pertinent seminars, bring them to the attention of your supervisor. Continued interest in learning new techniques highlights you as a possible candidate for a higher position or pay schedule. Medical employers will often pay tuition for seminars or classes.

Depending on what you need to learn, local adult education programs, community colleges, universities, and professional organizations all offer courses in the the skills required for the medical office. Read as much as possible on recent developments in your field.

Professional Organizations. Join the professional organizations most closely related to your new position. Many such organizations publish magazines with articles on recent developments in their fields. Professional organizations also hold regular local, regional, and national meetings with expert speakers. Such meetings also give you a chance to interact with others in your field and to share experiences. A list of professional organizations for medical office workers is included in the Appendix of this manual.

Move Ahead with the Organization. As your organization grows, it will become more professional, more up-to-date, and more sophisticated. It is important that you grow with your organization. Sometimes this requires considering new ideas or new possibilities.

Join the office team. Complete all tasks by the deadlines assigned, even if it means working later than usual. Be positive and cheerful in your dealings with other medical office workers and volunteer to assist co-workers on high-priority projects. In times of stress, remain courteous.

Demonstrate your ability to work independently by looking for ways to prevent problems, by taking the initiative to follow each task through to completion, and by organizing your work efficiently.

Always keep your goals in mind. Remember to model your actions, your behavior, your work, and your dress on those presently holding the position you want to achieve.

Follow these suggestions and you'll soon find yourself moving up the medical career ladder. Always do the best you can on each task and your efforts will be recognized. Best of luck!

Medical Ethics and Medical Law

LEGAL AND ETHICAL GUIDELINES

Medical ethics has been an important issue in the study of medicine since the Greek physician, Hippocrates, wrote his famous Hippocratic oath in 400 B.C. Today, the American Medical Association (AMA) provides leadership in addressing ethical issues in medicine for the United States, while similar organizations provide leadership in other countries. Physicians who are members of the AMA are bound by a *Code of Ethics* which focuses on (1) responsibility to the patient, (2) responsibility to society, (3) responsibility to others in the health care profession, and (4) responsibility to self. A physician's unethical behavior, while not always illegal, can result in censure and expulsion from the AMA.

Physicians can be imprisoned if they violate the laws that regulate their professional behavior. Two major precepts of medical law deal with (1) protection of the patient/physician relationship and (2) accountability to society. Since medical ethics and medical law often concern the same issues, it is not always possible to separate the two.

2.1 Comparison of Ethics and Law

Medical ethics is concerned with whether a physician's actions are right or wrong, while *medical law* is confined to whether the physician's actions are legal or illegal. *Ethical behavior*, according to the American Medical Association Judicial Council, refers to (1) moral principles and practices, (2) the customs and usages of the medical profession, and (3) matters of medical policy. The word *unethical* is used to describe behavior which fails to conform to ethical standards. When a physician has been accused of unethical conduct, the AMA Judicial Council has the authority to dismiss the accusation, to issue a warning or criticism, or to expel the physician from the Association.

The AMA does not have the authority to bring legal action against a member for unethical behavior.

Federal, state, and local laws govern the legal conduct of physicians, and a physician who is suspected of violating the law is subject to civil or criminal prosecution. If found guilty, the physician's medical license can be taken away, and the physician can be imprisoned. Often, a physician who is found guilty under the law is also censured by or expelled from the AMA or the local medical society. On the other hand, a physician who is acquitted by a court of law may still face disciplinary action from a medical society. The standards of medical ethics are often more strict than standards set by law, but they are never less strict.

2.2 AMA Principles of Medical Ethics/AAMA Code of Ethics

The American Medical Association and the American Association of Medical Assistants (AAMA) have adopted codes of ethics which provide guidelines for the professional behavior of physicians and medical assistants. Although the codes for the two organizations are different, they share important standards which everyone who works in a medical office should follow. Both codes speak of human dignity, confidentiality, continued study, and responsibility to society. With the permission of the AMA, the 1980 revision of the *Principles of Medical Ethics* is given below. The AAMA has also given permission to reprint its *Code of Ethics* directed to medical assistants.

AMA PRINCIPLES OF MEDICAL ETHICS	AAMA CODE OF ETHICS
Preamble:	**Preamble:**
The medical profession has long subscribed to a body of ethical statements developed primarily for the benefit of the patient. As a member of this profession, a physician must recognize responsibility not only to patients, but also to society, to other health professionals, and to self. The following principles adopted by the American Medical Association are not laws, but standards of conduct which define the essentials of honorable behavior for the physician.	The Code of Ethics of AAMA shall set forth principles of ethical and moral conduct as they relate to the medical profession and the particular practice of medical assisting. Members of AAMA dedicated to the conscientious pursuit of their profession, and thus desiring to merit the high regard of the entire medical profession and the respect of the general public which they serve, do pledge themselves to strive always to:

AMA (Continued)

Human Dignity

I. A physician shall be dedicated to providing competent medical service with compassion and respect for human dignity.

Honesty

II. A physician shall deal honestly with patients and colleagues, and strive to expose those physicians deficient in character or competence, or who engage in fraud or deception.

Responsibility to Society

III. A physician shall respect the law and recognize a responsibility to seek changes in those requirements which are contrary to the best interests of the patient.

Confidentiality

IV. A physician shall respect the rights of patients, of colleagues, and of other health professionals, and shall safeguard patient confidence within the constraints of the law.

Continued Study

V. A physician shall continue to study, apply and advance scientific knowledge, make relevant information available to patients, colleagues, and the public, obtain consultation, and use the talents of other health professionals where needed.

Freedom of Choice

VI. A physician shall, in the provision of appropriate patient care, except in emergencies, be free to choose whom to serve, with whom

AAMA (Continued)

Human Dignity

a. Render service with full respect for the dignity of humanity;

Confidentiality

b. Respect confidential information obtained through employment unless legally authorized or required by responsible performance of duty to divulge such information;

Honor

c. Uphold the honor and high principles of the profession and accept its disciplines;

Continued Study

d. Seek to continually improve the knowledge and skills of medical assistants for the benefit of patients and professional colleagues;

AMA (Continued)	AAMA (Continued)
to associate, and the environment in which to provide medical services.	
Responsibility to Improved Community	**Responsibility for Improved Community**
VII. A physician shall recognize a responsibility to participate in activities contributing to an improved community.	e. Participate in additional service activities aimed toward improving the health and well-being of the community.

2.3 Bioethics

The term *bioethics* refers to the branch of ethics which is concerned with moral issues resulting from high technology and sophisticated medical research. Social issues such as abortion, fetal research, artificial insemination, and euthanasia are important bioethical questions. In *Current Opinions of the Judicial Council*, the AMA states its position on 17 bioethical questions.

2.4 Licensure

Physicians may practice medicine only after they have met the legal requirements of the state in which they want to practice. Once all requirements are satisfied, the state issues a license which the doctor must renew periodically. Two of the medical office employee's important responsibilities are to maintain a record of the physician's license renewal date and to remind the doctor to renew the license at the appropriate time. The medical license can be revoked if a physician is convicted of a crime, engages in unprofessional conduct, or is mentally or physically disabled. Registered nurses (R.N.s), licensed practical nurses (L.P.N.s), and certain other medical professionals must also maintain current licenses. These licenses can also be revoked for unprofessional or illegal conduct.

2.5 Privilege of Patient Confidentiality

The law protects the patient's right of confidentiality, which means that medical offices, hospitals, and other health care facilities are legally bound to keep all patient information confidential. This concept, called *privilege of patient confidentiality*, assures individuals of the complete privacy of their records since it requires their written permission before any information can be released. When information is released, it should be provided by the physician only, except for insurance forms, which the medical secretary completes with the doctor's approval. Insurance forms have a statement of permission which the patient signs, granting the medical office the authority to release information to the insurance company (see Figure 2-1). Hospitals must also have written permission before releasing information (see Figure 2-2). The physician or medical office employee who releases confidential information without permission can be prosecuted.

Many doctors consider confidentiality to be the most desirable character trait that a medical office employee can have. In addition to moral concerns for confidentiality, physicians are legally responsible for the actions of their employees during the course of duty and can be sued if an employee releases confidential information.

Sometimes a husband, wife, friend, child, or employer of a patient may ask about the patient's condition. While these questions may come from a concerned individual, you should never provide information about the patient. Instead, refer the inquiry to the physician.

Wife: This is my husband's third heart attack. Do you think he can continue to work?

Medical Office Employee: I'm sorry, but I'm not qualified to give you that information. However, I would be happy to ask the doctor to talk with you.

Employer: My employee, Joseph Rankin, has missed work for three weeks because of a sore foot. Is his injury really that bad, or could he come back to work?

Medical Office Employee: I'm sorry but I will have to let the doctor answer that question. If you will leave your number, I will have Dr. Sparks call you.

Insurance Representative: Hello, my name is Virginia Wiley and I represent the United States Insurance Company. I have a question about the medical condition of our policyholder, Peter D'Angeleno.

Medical Office Employee: I'm sorry, but I can't release any information without the written consent of our patient. If you will mail us a patient consent form, I will see that you get the information you need.

Chapter 2—Medical Ethics and Medical Law 23

Figure 2-1 Permission to Release Information to Insurance Company

---

Stone Mountain General Insurance Company
158 Peachtree Street
Atlanta, GA 30304-1107

PATIENT & INSURED (SUBSCRIBER) INFORMATION		
1. PATIENT'S NAME *(First name, middle initial, last name)* Ellen V. Carson	2. PATIENT'S DATE OF BIRTH 8 | 15 | --	3. INSURED'S NAME *(First name, middle initial, last name)* Ellen V. Carson
4. PATIENT'S ADDRESS *(Street, city, state, ZIP code)* 5168 Oak Grove Terrace Atlanta, GA 30304-5475	5. PATIENT'S SEX MALE [ ] FEMALE [X] 7. PATIENT'S RELATIONSHIP TO INSURED SELF [X] SPOUSE [ ] CHILD [ ] OTHER [ ]	6. INSURED'S I.D. No. *(Including any letters)* 283-58-6871 8. INSURED'S GROUP No. *(Or Group Name)* TN 75281
9. OTHER HEALTH INSURANCE COVERAGE. Enter Name of Policyholder, Plan Name, Address and Policy. None	10. WAS CONDITION RELATED TO: A. PATIENT'S EMPLOYMENT YES [ ] NO [X] B. AN AUTO ACCIDENT YES [ ] NO [X]	11. INSURED'S ADDRESS *(Street, city, state, ZIP code)* 5168 Oak Grove Terrace Atlanta, GA 30304-5475
12. PATIENT'S OR AUTHORIZED PERSON'S SIGNATURE I hereby authorize the release of any medical information necessary to process this claim and request payment of benefits either to myself or to the party who accepts assignment below. SIGNATURE DATE		13. I authorize payment of medical benefits to undersigned physician or supplier for services described below. SIGNATURE (Insured or Authorized Person)

PHYSICIAN OR SUPPLIER INFORMATION		
14. DATE OF: 2/15/--	ILLNESS (FIRST SYMPTOM) OR INJURY (ACCIDENT) OR PREGNANCY (LMP)	15. DATE FIRST CONSULTED YOU FOR THIS CONDITION 4/14/--	16. HAS PATIENT EVER HAD SAME OR SIMILAR SYMPTOMS? YES [X] NO [ ]
17. DATE PATIENT ABLE TO RETURN TO WORK Immediately	18. DATES OF TOTAL DISABILITY FROM THROUGH	DATES OF PARTIAL DISABILITY FROM THROUGH
19. NAME OF REFERRING PHYSICIAN Jean Kirkpatrick, M.D.		20. FOR SERVICES RELATED TO HOSPITALIZATION GIVE HOSPITALIZATION DATES ADMITTED DISCHARGED
21. NAME & ADDRESS OF FACILITY WHERE SERVICES RENDERED *(If other than home or office)*		22. WAS LABORATORY WORK PERFORMED OUTSIDE YOUR OFFICE? YES [ ] NO [X] CHARGES

23. DIAGNOSIS OR NATURE OF ILLNESS OR INJURY, RELATE DIAGNOSIS TO PROCEDURE IN COLUMN D BY REFERENCE TO NUMBERS 1, 2, 3, ETC. OR DX CODE

1. Unstable arteriosclerotic heart disease, old myocardial infarction, and recent heart irregularity
2. Type II hyperglycemia
3. Essential hypertension

24. A DATE OF SERVICE	B.* PLACE OF SER. VICE	C. FULLY DESCRIBE PROCEDURES, MEDICAL SERVICE OR SUPPLIES FURNISHED FOR EACH DATE GIVEN		D DIAGNOSIS CODE	E CHARGES	DO NOT USE THIS AREA PAYMENT | DAYS
		PROCEDURE CODE IDENTIFY	*(EXPLAIN UNUSUAL SERVICES OR CIRCUMSTANCES)*			
4/14/--	3	90060	Routine office visit	1,2,3	25.00	
4/14/--	3	71020	Chest X ray	1	30.00	
4/14/--	3	93000	Electrocardiogram	1	30.00	
4/14/--	3	80003	Blood sugar check, 2 hr.	2	15.00	

25. SIGNATURE OF PHYSICIAN OR SUPPLIER *(Read below before signing)***	26. ACCEPT ASSIGNMENT YES [X] NO [ ]	27. TOTAL CHARGE 100.00	28. PROVIDER CODE 3458-A	29. PYMT CODE 100.00
	30. YOUR SOCIAL SECURITY NO. 328-54-1345	31. PHYSICIAN OR SUPPLIER'S NAME, ADDRESS, ZIP CODE AND TELEPHONE NO. John H. Sparks, M.D. 8504 Capricorn Drive Atlanta, GA 30033-7775		
32. YOUR PATIENT'S ACCOUNT NUMBER 839	33. YOUR EMPLOYER I.D. NO. 2083999022			

*PLACE OF SERVICE CODES
1. INPATIENT 2. OUTPATIENT 3. OFFICE 4. HOME
**I, A DULY LICENSED DOCTOR OF MEDICINE IN ACTIVE PRACTICE, CERTIFY THAT I PERSONALLY PERFORMED THE ABOVE SERVICES OR THE SERVICES WERE PERFORMED UNDER MY PERSONAL OBSERVATION, DIRECTION, AND SUPERVISION.

CF-002 (10-76)

Figure 2-2 Permission for Hospital to Release Information

Metropolitan Hospital
700 Linwood Place
Atlanta, GA 30304-7705

I, the undersigned, hereby authorize Metropolitan Hospital to release the following information from my (or give relationship _____) medical record. This authorization includes release of information concerning treatment of drug or alcohol abuse, drug-related conditions, alcoholism, and/or psychiatric/psychological conditions. Review of the records is also authorized.

The following information may be released or reviewed:

- (✓) Discharge Summary
- (✓) Face Sheet with Final Diagnosis
- ( ) Complications and Operative Procedures
- (✓) History and Physical
- (✓) Consultation Report(s)
- ( ) Operative Report(s) and Findings
- (✓) Reports of Tests and X rays
- (✓) Emergency Treatment(s)
- ( ) Out-patient Clinic Notes (Specify Clinic _____)
- ( ) Immunization (Shot) Records
- ( ) Other

Dates of Treatment 12/3/-- – 6/23/-- or Particular Illness (specify) _____

- (✓) In-patient
- ( ) Out-patient
- ( ) Emergency Dept.

The above information is to be forwarded to:

Name and Title of Person Dr. Abner Dowarksik
Agency/Hospital National Alcoholism Center
Street Address 128 Peachtree Street
City, State, and Zip Code Atlanta, GA 30304-7743

The above information is requested to be released for the following purpose only. Redisclosure requires separate written authorization. Treatment of chronic alcoholism

This statement must be signed and dated, and may be revoked at any time except to the extent action has been taken prior to revocation. This consent will expire in sixty (60) days after the date below, or sooner by my choice, in which case this consent will expire on _____ .

I hereby state that I have read and fully understand the above statements as they apply to me. I hereby consent to the disclosure of the treatment records to the purpose and extent stated above.

Patient's Name Mason Nadman
Address 5673 B Arline Lane
Atlanta, GA 30304-8792
Birthdate 6/18/34
Medical Record # 2345-56

Signature (of patient) *Mason Nadman*
Witness _____
Date May 14, 19--

*Patient is unable to sign because he/she is an unemancipated minor, _____ years of age, or for the following reason: _____

Witness: _____
Closest Relative or Legal Guardian _____

Chapter 2—Medical Ethics and Medical Law   25

2.6 Exception to Physician/Patient Privilege

The law protects society by requiring physicians to report certain situations and events to the authorities. This concept is called *exception to the physician/patient privilege*. Births, deaths, and crimes against individuals such as gunshot wounds and stabbings are examples of occurrences that a physician is *required* to report. If a crime appears to have been committed against a patient, the doctor is expected to alert the authorities and to provide information that would help to solve the crime. The medical office employee who suspects child abuse, rape, poisoning, or any other physical crime should inform the doctor immediately.

2.7 Patient Inquiries

Patients sometimes want more information than the physician is willing to give them without having performed further tests or additional treatment. In such cases, patients often ask the medical office employees about their conditions. Since you are not medically licensed, you are prohibited from discussing any medical details with the patient. When a patient asks such questions, politely decline to answer and refer the patient to the physician.

Patient: I have to come back for another pregnancy test. What did my first test show?

Medical Office Employee: Why don't I ask the doctor to talk to you again. She will be able to give you the results.

Patient: I've had the flu for a long time. Shouldn't it have cleared up by now? Do you think I'm taking the right medication?

Medical Office Employee: Why don't you ask the doctor what she thinks about that. I'm sure she will be glad to talk to you again.

2.8 Personal Information About Patients

Patients supply personal information about themselves for their records. Even though this information is not medical in nature, it is confidential and should not be released or discussed with anyone outside the office.

Friend: How old is Mrs. Geers? Does she have children?

Medical Office Employee: I really don't know, but even if I knew I couldn't tell you because it would be confidential information about one of our patients.

2.9 Releasing Information Inadvertently

Information in patient files can be released inadvertently by an individual who sees no harm in mentioning a personal or medical fact about a patient to a close friend. Carelessly released information can cause ethical and legal problems for the doctor and, consequently, for the individual who released it.

A good rule to follow is: Never talk about patients outside the medical office.

Friend: I saw the mayor in your office when I came to meet you for lunch. Is he sick?

Incorrect Response

Medical Office Employee: Don't say anything about this, but he's been in several times recently. We can't seem to regulate his diabetes medication.

Correct Response

Medical Office Employee: I'm sorry I can't talk about it, but you know I cannot discuss patients, even with my best friend!

2.10 Confidential Information About the Doctor

The physician is the only individual who should release personal information or information about the medical practice. Questions such as "How many patients does the doctor have?" "What is the rent on this building?" or "How much did the new CAT scan cost?" should be ignored or answered, "I'm not sure. You may want to ask the doctor about that."

MEDICAL MALPRACTICE/PROFESSIONAL LIABILITY

2.11 Malpractice Claims

A patient who thinks that a physician has been negligent in diagnosing and treating an illness or accident may file a medical malpractice claim. If a medical malpractice claim is proved, the physician or the physician's insurance company may have to pay hundreds of thousands of dollars in damages. According to the AMA's report, *Professional Liability in the 80s*,* 16 malpractice claims were filed in 1983 for every 100 doctors, with the current number of claims doubling the number filed ten years ago. While most medical malpractice claims are made against physicians, malpractice can also be claimed against others who work in medical offices or related health care facilities, including nurses, laboratory technicians, medical assistants, and medical secretaries. Claims against medical employees will be discussed further in Section 2.13, Rule of Personal Liability.

Basic to any medical malpractice claim is the belief that a health care professional failed to meet the standard of care considered normal in the patient's geographic area; and as a result, some harm was done to the person. This concept is called *negligence*. Patients must prove that a physician or other health care professional was negligent and failed to meet the standard of care that another physician or health care professional would have met in the same circumstances. Negligence may be claimed when a procedure is performed incorrectly or when an improper diagnosis is made. Patients may also claim negligence when their condition warrants the advice of a specialist and their physician does not seek such advice.

A patient may claim negligence or gross negligence (a high degree of negligence). The physician may assert a defense of contributory or comparative negligence on the part of the patient. The following cases are examples of negligence.

Negligence Case 1

An orthopedist failed to treat a hairline fracture in the ankle of a college football player. The doctor told the football player that he could continue to run on his ankle, as long as he took it easy. During a game, the player fell, shattering the ankle, and causing an exten-

---

Professional Liability in the 80s (Chicago: American Medical Association, 1984).

sive muscle tear. As a result, the football player was unable to meet the terms of a professional football contract he expected to sign. (Negligence)

Negligence Case 2

A physician failed to diagnose appendicitis when an adult complained of pain in her right side and gave other standard symptoms of appendicitis over a ten-day period. The physician did not order the usual laboratory tests and did not consider exploratory surgery. As a result, the appendix ruptured and the patient almost died. (Gross negligence)

2.12 Physician's Responsibility for Employees

Physicians are liable for the actions of their medical employees while the employees are on duty. The following case shows how a physician might be sued for malpractice based on the negligence of an employee.

Negligence Case 3

A medical assistant switched the urine samples of two patients by mistake. A patient diagnosed as healthy later went into diabetic coma because her diabetes had gone undiagnosed. The healthy patient suffered severe mental anguish and underwent treatment for diabetes unnecessarily.

2.13 Rule of Personal Liability

All individuals are held responsible for their own conduct. This means that a medical office employee can be held personally liable or jointly liable for medical malpractice. You, and other individuals who work with medications or with patients, are especially vulnerable to malpractice claims because you can be charged with practicing medicine without a license. Never leave the impression that you are recommending a treatment or a medication: a patient may interpret the comments of a medical office employee incorrectly and later charge the employee with practicing medicine illegally.

A medical office employee is responsible for reporting illegal acts performed by a physician. For example, when a doctor performs an illegal abortion, the medical office employee can be held jointly liable for the crime. Since physicians are required by law to report crimes they learn about through the practice of medicine, the medical office employee who knows of an unreported crime, such as a shooting or a stabbing, can be held jointly liable.

In today's society, the illegal use of drugs and the illegal prescription of drugs are concerns for medical office personnel. If you are knowingly involved in the illegal use or prescription of drugs, you can be held criminally responsible.

Engaging in sexual acts with patients who are under the influence of anesthesia is against the law. The medical office employee who commits a sexual aggression against a patient or who fails to report a sexual crime by the physician or another employee may be prosecuted.

Most professional liability policies allow employees to be covered for malpractice under the physician's policy. Ultimately, however, you are responsible for yourself and should carry your own liability insurance, even though you may also be covered under the physician's policy. By purchasing your own liability insurance, you can be sure that it never lapses due to a change of jobs, illness, or failure of the doctor to make an insurance payment on time. Even though malpractice or personal liability insurance is expensive for physicians, it is usually very reasonable for other health care professionals.

2.14   Preventing Malpractice Claims

The best way to protect against medical malpractice claims is to avoid situations which can result in malpractice. The most important preventive measure is maintenance of a complete medical record for each patient. Since medical records can be used as evidence during a malpractice court proceeding, they should be complete, accurate, and up-to-date at all times. They should include permissions to release information, permissions for surgery and other medical procedures, copies of all laboratory reports, a list of all medications prescribed and dispensed, the doctor's and nurse's notes, miscellaneous medical information, and a physician withdrawal form if the physician no longer treats the patient. Medicare and Medicaid records and records of other government-funded medical programs should also be included.

The medical office employee has a responsibility to the physician, to patients, and to self to prevent medical malpractice claims. A malpractice suit can destroy the practice of a respected physician or other health care professional.

2.15   Patient Consent

A patient may consent to procedures for diagnosis and treatment and thus relieve the physician of liability. A consent form for each specific medical situation requiring consent should be prepared for the patient's signature before the procedure is begun. The reason for the

Figure 2-3 Consent Form

ACKNOWLEDGEMENT OF INFORMED CONSENT
FOR SURGICAL OR MEDICAL PROCEDURES

I hereby indicate that I have given consent to _____Dr. John Sparks_____ (insert doctor's name), with associates or assistants of his choice, to perform the following surgical, diagnostic, and or medical procedure (including without limit anesthesia, X rays, or laboratory tests on ~~myself~~ Martin Lashley, Jr. my _____son_____ (cross out inappropriate description of patient):

_____Appendectomy_____

NAME OF PROCEDURE(S)

I hereby indicate that in giving this consent the nature and purpose of the procedure; what the procedure is expected to accomplish; alternate means of therapy, if any; and reasonably known risks, complications, and discomfort have been explained to me by the above named doctor.

I understand that during the course of the above described procedure, unforeseen conditions may be revealed that make advisable an extension of this procedure or the use of a different procedure. I hereby authorize the above named doctor(s) to carry out any extension or to perform any other procedure that in the doctor's judgement is advisable for my well being if circumstances make it impossible or, in the doctor's opinion, medically undesirable, to obtain my specific consent to such extension or other procedure. The authority granted under this paragraph shall extend to treating all conditions that require treatment and are not known to the above named doctors at the time the procedure is commenced.

I am aware that the practice of medicine and surgery is not an exact science and that the possibility and nature of results or complications cannot be anticipated with complete accuracy. I acknowledge that no guarantees, express or implied, have been made as to the results of the above described procedure or any cure.

I consent to the admittance of observers and to the photographing or televising of the surgical, diagnostic, and or medical procedure to be performed, including appropriate portions of my body provided my name or identity is not revealed by the pictures or by the descriptive texts accompanying them.

Date ___May 18, 19--___
Time ___8___ (a.m.)/p.m.

_____WITNESS_____

SIGNATURE OF PATIENT

___Betsy Lashley___
SIGNATURE OF PARENT (WHERE REQUIRED)

SIGNATURE OF OTHER PERSON WITH LEGAL AUTHORITY (WHERE REQUIRED)

consent, plus any risks, should be explained in detail to the patient. Patient consent is required before surgery, before an experimental procedure is performed, before experimental drugs are used, and before other related procedures are undertaken.

2.16 Malpractice or Professional Liability Insurance

A physician who is sued for medical malpractice can expect the litigation to be lengthy and expensive. Costs will at least include court fees and attorney fees if the case is won, and if the case is lost, a monetary award to the patient must be added. These costs can run into hundreds of thousands, even millions, of dollars. Since few physicians are able to pay all the expenses of a malpractice suit through personal funds, malpractice or professional liability insurance is available. The insurance is very expensive, but the expense is minor compared to the amount that will be paid if a physician is found guilty of malpractice.

If a physician is sued, a Summons and Complaint will be received through the mail or will be hand delivered by the sheriff's department. These legal documents should be brought to the physician's attention immediately. Failure to promptly respond could result in a default judgment; that is, a judgment against the physician because no answer was made.

2.17 Malpractice Lawsuits

A patient who believes that a physician is guilty of negligence can sue for medical malpractice. The patient, who is the plaintiff in a malpractice suit, must prove that the physician was negligent; the physician, who is the defendant, must show that the plaintiff's accusation is false. The burden of proof in a malpractice suit is therefore on the plaintiff. Since proving innocence requires excellent medical records, the importance of the medical office employee's record-keeping system becomes clear. Some malpractice lawsuits last for months or years and require extensive review of the physician's medical records.

When a malpractice claim is made against a physician or other health care professional, the person against whom the claim is made reports it to the insurance company carrying the professional liability coverage. The insurance company then hires an attorney to defend the physician or health care professional. The attorney reviews the patient's medical records and talks with the patient, the physician, the medical office employees, and others who might have information important to the case. Then, after all the facts have been gathered, the attorney answers the patient's charge through legal documents presented to the court.

2.18 Depositions

A *deposition* is a sworn statement given by a party to a lawsuit before the suit goes to trial. During a deposition, an attorney asks questions of an individual. The answers are recorded by a stenographer or court reporter who takes the statement in shorthand or by machine, types the document in final form, and notarizes it. As a medical office employee, you may be asked to give a deposition. If so, tell the complete facts as you know them, without changing them in any way. If you are unsure of your answers, say so.

2.19 Settlement of a Malpractice Lawsuit

Many malpractice lawsuits never go to trial because the physician's insurance company and the patient's attorney agree on a dollar amount of damages to be paid to the patient before trial. Usually the patient's attorney makes a dollar demand of the attorney representing the insurance company, and the insurance company's attorney responds with a counteroffer. This process can continue for several months. Once all parties to the lawsuit agree on a damage figure, a settlement is made and the physician's insurance company pays the patient. Some cases go to trial before a settlement is reached, and a settlement is made during the trial. Most medical malpractice policies require the physician's consent to a proposed settlement. The court may also dismiss the suit for failure of the plaintiff to establish a cause of action against the doctor. This means that the patient does not have a good enough argument against the doctor.

2.20 Medical Malpractice Trials

When a physician and the physician's professional liability insurance carrier feel that no malpractice took place or cannot agree with the plaintiff on a settlement, the case goes to trial. During the trial, testimony is given by the parties involved in the lawsuit. After all the evidence is presented to the court, a judge or a jury decides the physician's innocence or guilt. If the physician is found guilty, monetary damages are set by the judge or jury, and the malpractice carrier pays the patient up to the limits set by the physician's insurance policy. The physician must personally pay any difference between the policy limit and the damages set by the judge or jury.

2.21 Good Samaritan Laws

Emergencies occur which can result in death if a physician or other health care professional "on the scene" does not offer treatment. Such emergencies include automobile accidents, people choking at restaurants, and similar events. Good Samaritan laws in all 50 states encourage physicians to offer treatment without fear of a malpractice suit. Generally, these laws cover the physician and other health care professionals who provide treatment within their areas of expertise. However, the laws in each state are different, so check the law in your state to determine the extent of professional liability during an emergency.

CONTROLLED SUBSTANCES ACT

2.22 Dispensing Drugs

The Controlled Substances Act governs the use of drugs in medical offices. Because of the high potential for drug abuse in our society, physicians who dispense narcotic drugs are required to maintain complete and detailed records. Physicians who keep only nonnarcotic drugs in their offices are not required to maintain detailed records. If you are responsible for maintaining the drug records in your office, include the following information in the drug file:

- Name and address of all patients to whom a drug was given
- Date, name, and quantity of drug given
- Dispensing method
- Reason drug was given

2.23 Prescribing Drugs

Only a physician has the authority to prescribe controlled substances. However, with the physician's permission, a medical office employee may phone some prescriptions for controlled substances to the pharmacy.

2.24 Drug Schedules

Drugs are divided into five categories or schedules, depending on their potential for abuse. The drug schedules and examples of drugs falling into each category are listed below:

Schedule I. Drugs listed in Schedule I have a high potential for abuse. They are not legitimately used for treating patients in the United States, but with special permission Schedule I drugs may be used for research. Examples: heroin, LSD, peyote, mescaline, and PCP.

Schedule II. Schedule II drugs have a high potential for abuse and may lead to psychological or physical dependence. They have been accepted for medical use in the United States. Schedule II drugs can only be dispensed with a prescription signed by a physician; no telephone prescriptions are acceptable. Examples: Percodan, morphine, codeine, Dilaudid, methadone, cocaine, Seconal, Nembutal, Amytal, and Quaalude.

Schedule III. The potential for abuse is lessened with Schedule III drugs. Though use of the drugs is accepted in the United States, a moderate degree of physical or psychological dependence may result from abuse. Schedule III drugs can be dispensed with a written prescription. The physician can order telephone refills of Schedule III drugs. Examples: Tylenol No. 3 with codeine, Empirin No. 3 with codeine, Fiorinal, Phenobarbital, Paregoric, Butisol and Noludar.

Schedule IV. Schedule IV drugs have low potential for abuse and have been accepted for medical use in the United States. Abuse may lead to limited physical or psychological dependence. Prescriptions for Schedule IV drugs may be written by someone other than a physician, as long as the physician signs the prescription. Refills can be approved by the medical office employee as long as the physician is consulted. Examples: Valium, Librium, Tranxene.

Schedule V. The potential for abuse of Schedule V drugs is low. These drugs are accepted for medical use in the United States and can be purchased without a prescription. Abuse may lead to a more limited physical or psychological dependence than will abuse of Schedule IV drugs. Examples: Donnagel PG, Novahistine DH, Novahistine Expectorant.

REFERENCES

American Association of Medical Assistants Bylaws, Chicago: American Association of Medical Assistants, 1984.

Current Opinions of the Judicial Council of the American Medical Association - 1984. Chicago: American Medical Association, 1984.

Bernzweig, E. P. *The Nurse's Liability for Malpractice: A Programmed Course,* 3d ed. New York: McGraw-Hill Book Company, 1981.

Bullough, B. (ed.). *The Law and the Expanding Nursing Role,* 2d ed. New York: Appleton-Century-Croft, 1980.

Frumer, L. R., *et al.* (eds.). *Personal Injury—Actions, Defenses, Damages.* 25 vols. New York: Matthew Bender, 1982.

Hemlet, M. D. and M. E. Mackert. *Dynamics of Law in Nursing and Health Care.* Reston, Virginia: Reston Publishing Company, Inc., 1978.

Lewis, M. and C. Warden. *Law and Ethics in the Medical Office Including Bioethical Issues.* Philadelphia: F. A. Davis Co., 1982.

Soukhanov, A. H. and J. R. Haverty. *Webster's Medical Office Handbook.* Springfield, Massachusetts: G. C. Merriam Company, 1979.

3

Interpersonal Skills

The first contact a patient has with the medical office usually involves verbal and nonverbal communications. This may be a greeting from the receptionist or medical secretary when the patient enters the office, or it may be a telephone conversation to schedule an appointment. The tone of your voice and your manner are important when you communicate with patients because they establish the type of relationship formed between the patient and the office.

Verbal communications are the oral messages an individual sends to others. They include face-to-face encounters, telephone conversations, instructions, speeches, oral reports, questions, off-hand remarks, and other forms of speaking. Good verbal communications depend on proper word usage and on nonverbal communications.

Nonverbal communications are gestures, facial expressions, tone of voice, appearance, and other unspoken messages that an individual sends. In a medical office, nonverbal messages are very important. A friendly smile can cheer a patient who has a lengthy wait. A concerned voice can soothe the mother of a sick child, and a professional manner can calm a hysterical patient. In general, a caring attitude can help relieve the stress of being sick.

When verbal and nonverbal communications fail to deliver the same message, patients become confused. They do not understand the message. The medical office employee who greets people with friendly words and an aloof manner makes them uncomfortable. The physician who asks questions but does not listen for answers alarms patients. Just as you are careful to use correct words when you speak, so should you be careful to send appropriate nonverbal messages.

HUMAN RELATIONS

Human relations skills are as important as office skills and should be developed with the same attention. Several human relations skills which are valuable for building good interpersonal relationships are discussed below.

3.1 Patience

People who are sick often behave in an unusual manner. They may be cranky and irritable or quiet and nervous. They need to be treated with understanding and patience. It is easy for the medical office employee to become impatient when the reception room is crowded, patients are irritable, and the doctor is behind schedule. Yet you must guard against impatience because it adds to patients' stress. When you are impatient, breathe deeply and relax. Do not allow your frustration to interfere with the way you interact with people.

Patient: I've been here 30 minutes. How much longer do I have to wait? I have other things to do today.

Incorrect Response

Medical Office Employee: Well, I'm sorry, but you shouldn't have made the appointment if you were on a tight schedule. Medical offices are busy places.

Correct Response

Medical Office Employee: I'm sorry, but we have had a delay. We had several emergencies this morning, and we've been trying to catch up since.

Patient: I've been coming to Dr. Sparks for ten years; but when I called for an appointment you made me wait three weeks to see the doctor. I don't think that is fair, and I'm going to complain.

Incorrect Response

Medical Office Employee: You should know that we can't give you an appointment any time you want. This is a busy office. You'll just have to wait until there is an opening.

Correct Response

Medical Office Employee: We're sorry you had to wait so long for an appointment. The last few weeks have been very busy, and we try not to overschedule. We will, of course, work you in immediately any time an emergency arises.

3.2 Poise

Poise goes hand in hand with patience. Being poised means keeping a cool head under pressure and remaining calm during hectic periods. People have different reasons for visiting the doctor. They come for routine checkups, because they are ill, and for emergencies. You should remain poised and self-assured in each situation. On some days, the office will run smoothly, the physician will stay on schedule, and all office employees will be at work. It is easy to remain poised on such days. On other days, several additional patients will need to be worked into an already busy schedule, the physician will fall behind, and one or more office workers will be out sick. On such days your poise will be tested severely. To remain poised, stay calm. Work methodically and as rapidly as possible, but do not rush. Advise patients of any unusual circumstances and ask for their understanding; then set aside any work which can wait until another day. Handle one task at a time and try not to allow yourself to feel pressured.

During emergencies, you must remain calm. An emergency patient or individuals accompanying an emergency patient may become hysterical and excite others in the reception room. Compose yourself and work efficiently, but do not rush.

Situation

In the middle of a busy day when several patients remain to be seen, a co-worker advises the medical office employee that she isn't feeling well and must leave.

Unpoised Reaction

The medical office employee tries to handle his own tasks, the co-worker's chores, and the patients. As a result, he becomes pressured and nervous and sends negative nonverbal messages to the patients and the physician. At the end of the day, the tension level in the office is high; the medical office employee is frustrated and unhappy.

Poised Reaction

The medical office employee asks his co-worker to make a list of all unfinished tasks which must be completed before the end of the day.

Any chores which can be delayed until the co-worker returns are set aside. When not attending to patients, the medical office employee handles one task at a time. At the end of the day, several tasks remain to be completed. The medical office employee stays late to finish those which cannot wait and makes a list of the others to give to his co-worker.

3.3 Sensitivity

A medical office employee must be sensitive to the physical and emotional concerns of all patients. This includes being aware of stressful situations and easing them when possible. Personal and medical questions about the patient's history should be asked diplomatically and professionally since some routine questions are embarrassing to patients. Questions should never be asked out of curiosity.

Sensitivity means that you are concerned about privacy. Make certain your conversations are never overheard by others. You should be aware that voices carry, so speak softly enough that patients in other examining rooms cannot hear you.

Some patients are sensitive about undressing and are embarrassed when they are asked to remove their clothes for an examination. You should give explicit directions regarding which clothes to remove, then leave the room while the patient undresses. Give the patient a gown or drape to wear during the examination.

Situation

A female teenager sees the doctor for a complete physical examination before beginning work as a camp counselor. She appears to be nervous when asked to undress.

Insensitive Reaction

Medical Office Employee: Please take off your clothes so the doctor can check you. Here's a gown (or drape).

Sensitive Reaction

Medical Office Employee: Please remove your blouse so the doctor can listen to your heart. You may leave your skirt on. Here's a gown (or drape) to cover your chest. I'll check back with you in a few minutes.

3.4 Friendliness

Patients respond best to a warm, caring personality. Even the patients who seem cold are relieved when the medical office staff is cordial. Friendliness is often transmitted in a nonverbal way, such as with a smile, a touch to the shoulder, a friendly nod, or a handshake. Always try to be friendly, even though you may feel tired or cross. While the busy routine of a medical office can make you forget the importance of a friendly smile, try not to appear aloof and uncaring.

3.5 Consideration

Consideration means thinking of others, both patients and co-workers. It includes slowing your pace for an elderly patient who is using a walker or a cane, checking back with patients when the physician is delayed, helping a co-worker when you are not busy, and volunteering to come to work early some days. Consideration and cooperation make an individual well-liked and respected.

DISPLAYING WORTHY CHARACTER TRAITS

Character traits are a form of nonverbal communication. They help others form an impression of an individual's values. Several character traits are important for a medical office employee. Some of them are discussed below.

3.6 Honesty

The honesty of medical office employees must be unquestionable. Because the physician can be held responsible for the actions of employees, honesty is an important element of the relationship between the doctor and the medical office employee. Drugs and the money from patient fees are likely targets of theft by dishonest individuals. Theft is not only immoral, it is a crime.

A dishonest person does not always commit a crime. Dishonesty may be in the form of a lie told to cover up a mistake, or it may involve counting too much overtime during a week in order to receive a larger paycheck. Dishonesty is a character flaw which will destroy a career as a medical office employee.

Dishonest Medical Office Employee: No, Dr. Sparks, I didn't break the stethoscope. Someone must have knocked it off the counter.

Honest Medical Office Employee: Yes, Dr. Sparks, I broke the stethoscope. I knocked it off the counter by accident.

3.7 Confidentiality

Confidentiality is a very desirable character trait for a medical office employee. In addition to the trust patients have in the doctor and the doctor's staff, the physician is legally bound to keep medical records confidential. Permission to release information is required from a patient before medical records can be discussed with anyone other than the patient (see Section 2.5, page 21).

3.8 Dependability

Dependability is among the most important character traits for a medical office employee. Because of the special nature of the office, you may receive little direct supervision. You must know what needs to be done, how to do it, which chores should be handled immediately, and which can wait. The physician depends on you to make the right decision, or to ask questions when you feel unqualified to make a decision. Dependable medical office employees get to work on time and finish work without being reminded. At times they stay after hours to complete work. Dependable office employees take sick leave only when sick and take the allotted amount of time for lunch each day.

3.9 Self-Confidence

The physician will not always be available to guide the activities of the medical office staff. It is important for the medical office employee to learn office procedures thoroughly and to feel confident about managing the office when the physician is unavailable. This means that when an emergency patient enters the office, emergency procedures are put into effect immediately and efficiently. It also means that the medical office assistant can answer the doctor's office questions quickly and confidently. Self-confidence is an important trait for anyone who works with patients. If the medical office employee is not confident about his or her ability and skill, patients will sense it and become nervous.

3.10 Flexibility

Flexibility is the ability to adjust your routine on a moment's notice. When an emergency occurs or the doctor needs something important, medical office employees need to respond without delay. Flexible people are able to do another employee's work when that person is out of the office. They come to work early or stay late, and rearrange lunch when necessary. When you are flexible, you are not set in a pattern that you cannot change.

Flexible Employee: Certainly, Dr. Sparks, I can help you now. I will file the patient folders later.

Inflexible Employee: Could you ask someone else to help you, Dr. Sparks? I need to file the patient folders.

3.11 Loyalty

A loyal medical office employee tactfully defends the physician when a patient complains about fees, services performed, or medicines prescribed. A loyal employee remains silent when other workers grumble about their salaries or their work and does not gossip about the physician's personal business or the practice. The physician deserves the loyalty of all the people who work in the medical office. An individual who does not respect the doctor should look for other employment.

3.12 Assertiveness

Assertiveness means speaking up when a comment needs to be made, or defending your position when appropriate. Assertiveness is sometimes confused with aggressiveness, but the terms have different meanings. *Aggressiveness* means being pushy or being the first to attack; sometimes it has a negative connotation. *Assertive* is a positive term which means to act on your own behalf, including making suggestions about office procedures, reminding the physician of a change in office procedures, and asking for a special privilege when it's important, such as asking permission to go home when you are ill.

Assertive Employee: Dr. Sparks, how long is the probationary period in this office? Will I receive an increase in pay at the end of the probation?

Aggressive Employee: Dr. Sparks, I've worked here three months. I think I deserve a raise.

3.13 Professionalism

Professionalism encompasses the way you look, the way you act, the language you use, and your attention to career growth. A professional refuses to gossip, dresses in an appropriate manner, wears a suitable hair style, and works with quiet confidence. Professional demeanor coupled with strong office skills leads to success in a medical office.

Unprofessional Employee	**Professional Employee**
Scuffed shoes	Polished shoes
Frayed collar	Neatly dressed
Long, swinging hair	Well-groomed hair, short or tied back
Heavy make-up	Subdued make-up
Coarse language	Appropriate language
Shrill voice	Calm, clear voice
Nonmember of professional organizations	Member of professional organizations
Silly, undignified manner	Dignified manner

GREETING PATIENTS AND OTHER VISITORS

3.14 Greeting Returning Patients

Greet patients immediately when they walk into the office. If you are busy with another task, stop long enough to say "Hello, Mr. Nozaki, I will be right with you." After greeting the patient, finish your task quickly or set it aside until later. If you are talking on the telephone, acknowledge the individual's presence with a friendly nod and a smile. Then finish your conversation as quickly as possible and give the visitor your full attention. A patient should never have to wait more than a minute before being greeted.

3.15 Greeting New Patients

Patients who have seen the physician before know the office routine, but new patients need more guidance. Give the new patient a pen or pencil and any forms which must be completed for the medical record. Explain the office's billing practices, payment methods, working hours, and after-hours emergency procedures. Mention the names of other doctors sharing the practice, and the names of the hospitals where the doctor is affiliated. When all preliminary forms have been completed, point out the magazines and tell the patient the doctor will be available soon.

Chapter 3—Interpersonal Skills 43

3.16   Greeting Visitors Other Than Patients

Salespersons, relatives of patients, representatives of civic organizations, the physician's attorney and stockbroker, and other visitors occasionally come to the medical office without an appointment. It is important to determine which visitors the doctor wishes to see. When possible, most physicians will see relatives of patients. Some will see salespeople offering innovative equipment or supplies. Others prefer the staff to screen all visitors and to preview equipment or supplies.

When the physician agrees to see unscheduled visitors, you must determine the nature of the visitor's business. A simple, "Good morning, may I help you?" is usually sufficient to obtain the names of visitors and the nature of their business. Sometimes it is necessary to ask, "May I tell the doctor why you are calling?" If the visitor is treated courteously, this information is usually freely given. If visitors refuse to state their names and reasons for calling, advise them that the doctor's schedule is full and that visitors are seen by appointment only. Be courteous even when refusing a request.

MAINTAINING THE RECEPTION AREA

The appearance of the reception area sends a nonverbal message to patients and other visitors. Magazines lying askew and cigarette butts in the ashtray make a negative statement about the office. They say that the physician and the office employees are sloppy and that they don't care about appearances. A patient might think that this lack of concern for details carries over to the treatment of patients.

3.17   Setting Up the Reception Area

Each evening you should arrange the waiting room for the next day. Place magazines in a rack or on tables so patients can find them, and water and dust plants. If visitors are allowed to smoke in the reception area, empty the ashtrays. If chairs have been moved during the day, move them to their correct positions. If these chores are handled by a cleaning crew, simply leave a note regarding any special tasks.

3.18   Routine Reception Area Maintenance

The reception area carpet should be vacuumed and the windows should be cleaned several times a week. The area should be dusted and given a good general cleaning as well. These jobs are usually handled by the cleaning staff under the medical office employee's supervision.

Medical Communications

HANDLING EMERGENCIES

You should always be prepared for an emergency in a medical office. Be aware of the proper procedures for handling emergencies, and with poise and confidence you will manage even the most difficult situations.

3.19 Walk-in Emergencies

Walk-in emergencies always alter the office routine and cause confusion because the emergency patient must see the doctor immediately. In an emergency, a medical office employee must be confident and self-assured because the patient, people accompanying the patient, and those waiting in the reception area will be tense and anxious. You must be calm and efficient: the patient's health depends on it.

As soon as the walk-in emergency patient appears, alert the doctor and take the person to an examining room; then alert your co-workers who may need to assist the doctor. Take anyone who accompanies the emergency victim to a different room, so they will not interfere with the doctor's examination. Assure them that the patient will receive the best of care. Advise patients in the reception area of the delay as soon as you can and schedule new appointments if necessary.

If the physician is not in the office at the time of an emergency, take the patient to an examining room and alert the nurse. If the nurse thinks that the patient should go to a hospital, call an ambulance to transport the patient. Locate the doctor and give a full description of the patient's problem and the name of the hospital to which the patient was transferred.

3.20 Call-in Emergencies

Emergency calls are disruptive to the office routine because they have top priority over other activities taking place in the medical office. These calls represent serious, sometimes life-threatening situations for patients.

Calming the Caller. People who place emergency calls are often nervous and agitated, sometimes hysterical; therefore, you must keep calm during an emergency in order to calm the caller. Several attempts at reassurance may be necessary before the caller is able to give important information about the emergency victim.

The best way to calm an agitated person is to ask for the facts of the emergency. If the caller is impossible to calm, ask for another person who can give the facts of the emergency.

First Call

Caller: A car just ran a stop sign and hit a woman who was walking down the street.

Medical Office Employee: Have you called the police?

Caller: No, but the doctor needs to come right away.

Medical Office Employee: Tell me the location of the accident, and I will call the police who will arrange medical help.

Caller: Will the doctor come?

Medical Office Employee: Did the woman ask for Dr. Sparks?

Caller: No, but I went to Dr. Sparks one time, and he's the only doctor I know.

Medical Office Employee: We're glad you called, but the woman may have a personal physician. I'll call the police who will contact the rescue unit. When the police arrive, they will ask the victim who her physician is or will call a relative if one is identified in her wallet. Please give me the location of the victim so I can call the police.

Second Call

Caller: I need to talk to the doctor. My husband is having a heart attack.

Medical Office Employee: Tell me your husband's symptoms.

Caller: I want to talk to the doctor!

Medical Office Employee: I am having someone get Dr. Sparks for you. But I need you to tell me your husband's symptoms.

Caller: Oh, he's getting worse!

Medical Office Employee: Is anyone else in the house?

Caller: My son-in-law.

Medical Office Employee: Would you please ask your son-in-law to come to the phone?

The conversation continues between the medical office employee and the son-in-law or between the doctor and the caller.

Getting Specific Information. Certain specific information is crucial in determining the severity of an emergency. This information includes:

1. The nature of the emergency (What happened?)
2. When the emergency occurred (How long ago?)
3. The extent of the emergency (How bad?)
4. Treatment provided (What has been done for the patient?)

After learning the details of an emergency, ask the physician whether the emergency patient should be brought to the office or transported directly to the hospital. If the physician is out of the office, ask the nurse. If both the physician and the nurse are unavailable, ask the patient to go directly to a hospital emergency room. Then call the emergency room to tell them that the patient is on the way. Then locate the physician and provide full details about the victim.

Arranging for Emergency Medical Care. When a caller reports a life-threatening emergency, you should arrange for immediate care. Life-threatening emergencies include heart attacks, poisonings, automobile accidents, gunshot wounds, and internal bleeding. After advising the physician of the emergency, call the police and give the patient's location. The dispatcher will send a rescue unit to the scene and will alert the emergency room that a patient is on the way. If the patient has experienced severe trauma, the rescue unit will go to the nearest hospital. Once the patient has stabilized, a private ambulance can transfer the patient to whatever hospital the physician designates.

4

Telephone Communication

The first impression people form of the medical office often is based on a telephone call. Your telephone manner and tone of voice are important factors in creating a good professional image for the office. Speak clearly and slowly and give full attention to the caller.

ANSWERING THE TELEPHONE

A ringing telephone should be answered as soon as possible: by the second ring at the latest. Patients may be irritable and demanding when they are ill, and a ringing telephone adds to the stress of both the caller and the people waiting to see the doctor.

4.1 Telephone Greetings

Several greetings are acceptable when answering the telephone in a medical office. If the practice includes only one or two physicians, their names may be included as a part of the greeting. In a large group practice, ''Doctor's office'' or the corporation's name, ''Medical Services,'' may eliminate the confusion caused by mentioning all the names. The words ''Good morning'' or ''Good afternoon'' and ''May I help you'' should be part of the greeting. It is not necessary to give the name of the individual answering the phone.

Use These Greetings: ''Good morning, Dr. Sparks's office. May I help you?''

''Good afternoon, Doctors' office. May I help you?''

Do Not Use This Greeting: ''Good morning, Doctors Sparks, Moore, Melville, Sanchez, and Robinson.''

4.2 Screening Calls

Some callers, both patients and nonpatients, ask for the doctor, even when someone else could handle the call adequately. If the physician talked to each of these people, no time would be left for examining patients. Therefore, screen all telephone calls and transfer them to the person who can best handle the caller's inquiry. Ask questions to clarify the reason the person is calling. Always ask the caller's name before transferring the call.

Appointments. Most people who telephone the medical office want to schedule an appointment. The receptionist usually handles these calls. If the patient asks for the physician and you suspect an appointment is needed, ask if you can schedule an appointment. Ask whether morning or afternoon is preferable; then make the arrangements for the earliest, most convenient date and time.

Medical Office Employee: Good morning, Dr. Sparks's office. May I help you?

Caller: I'd like to talk to Dr. Sparks.

Medical Office Employee: He's with a patient. May I help you?

Caller: I guess so. I'd like to come in to see the doctor.

Medical Office Employee: Would you like to come on August 4 in the morning or August 9 in the afternoon? (See Section 8.2, page 131).

Medical Conditions. Some calls from patients concern their medical condition or medication. These calls should be transferred to the nurse who will answer the question or check with the physician and call the patient back. If the nurse is not available, ask for the relevant facts to give to the physician.

Medical Office Employee: Good morning, Dr. Sparks's office. May I help you?

Caller: No, I need to talk to Dr. Sparks.

Medical Office Employee: He's with a patient at the moment. Will you leave a message?

Caller: I don't feel good. I think I may have the flu.

Medical Office Employee: What is your name, please?

Caller: Rose Corgan.

Medical Office Employee: Let me transfer you to the nurse, Mr. Mann. He can listen to your symptoms and ask Dr. Sparks to call you back. (See Section 4.5, page 52.)

Prescription Refills. Patients often call the medical office for a prescription refill or for medication. These calls can be handled by the person who answers the telephone. Gather all necessary information from the caller.

Medical Office Employee: Dr. Sparks's office. May I help you?

Caller: Dr. Sparks, please.

Medical Office Employee: Dr. Sparks is with a patient. May I help you?

Caller: No, I don't think so.

Medical Office Employee: Would you like to schedule an appointment?

Caller: No, I need my prescription refilled.

Medical Office Employee: I can take the information about your refill and call the drugstore with Dr. Sparks's permission. Then I will call and tell you what the doctor says.

Billing Charges and Insurance. Both patients and insurance representatives call the medical office to ask about fees charged for medical services. Frequently this information is needed for completion of an insurance form or to understand a charge. Remember, a medical office employee cannot legally release medical information to anyone without both the doctor's and the patient's permission. You must be careful to give only billing information when you discuss patient charges.

Medical Office Employee: Dr. Sparks's office. May I help you?

Caller: This is Lori Barrett from National Insurance Company. I would like information about your patient, Gladys Moncrief.

Medical Office Employee: How may I help you?

Caller: Her insurance claim form shows that she had a baby by cesarean section on July 4. Why was that necessary?

Medical Office Employee: I can't give you that information without the patient's authorizaton. Please send us a signed release and we will provide the appropriate information.

Test Results. Physicians frequently ask patients to call the office for test results. The medical office employee is usually given permission to inform patients of the results of minor tests. The physician informs patients of major test results.

Illness. In a few instances, the caller must talk to the physician directly and immediately. When screening a call, you must determine whether it should be transferred to the doctor, perhaps interrupting the examination of a patient, or whether it can wait until the doctor is free. If the call can wait, take the patient's number and give the approximate time when the doctor will telephone. Write a complete explanation of the reason for the call so the doctor will have background information. Put the message on the doctor's desk.

Related Calls. Other calls may be from salespeople, representatives of charity organizations, or civic leaders. The physician may wish to talk to some, but not all, of these individuals. Related calls often are difficult to screen because some callers say that the physician has asked to be telephoned or that the business is "personal." If callers will not leave a name or phone number, suggest that they write to the medical office. Remember, callers with legitimate business do not mind leaving their names. If you determine that the doctor would like to talk to the person, transfer the call. If the doctor is with a patient, take a message and telephone number for a return call. You should ask the physician which calls should be handled by the office staff and which calls the physician would like to handle personally.

Medical Office Employee: Dr. Sparks's office. May I help you?

Caller: Dr. Sparks, please.

Medical Office Employee: Dr. Sparks is with a patient. May I help you?

Chapter 4—Telephone Communication 51

Caller: No, this is a personal call.

Medical Office Employee: If you will leave your name and number, I will ask Dr. Sparks to return your call.

Caller: No thanks.

4.3 Taking General Messages

Eight pieces of information are needed for each telephone message taken for another person in the office. This information includes:

- The date of the call
- The time of the call
- The person called
- The caller's name
- The caller's telephone number
- Whether the caller will telephone again
- The complete message
- The initials of the person who took the call

Most medical offices use commercially prepared forms for recording telephone messages. When you complete a message, record all information clearly. After the problem has been handled, the message and the action taken are recorded in the patient's medical record.

Figure 4-1 Telephone Message Form

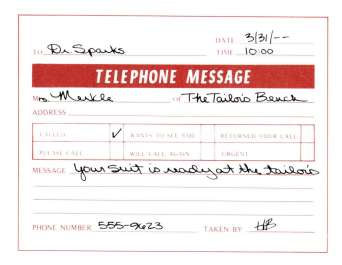

4.4 Taking Medical Messages

In some specialties, such as pediatrics and internal medicine, patients call to ask advice about a medical condition or to ask for approval of a prescription refill. When taking medical messages, it is important to get complete information. Ask clear, direct questions; when you are confident that you have all the information, tell the patient you will check with the physician and call back.

The following are questions to ask the caller regarding prescription refills:

1. The name of the patient
2. The name of the medication
3. How long the patient has taken the medication
4. The patient's symptoms
5. The patient's age and weight if a child
6. The name and telephone number of the pharmacy the patient uses
7. The patient's phone number

The following are questions to ask the caller regarding an illness:

1. The name of the sick patient
2. The patient's symptoms
3. When symptoms first appeared
4. Whether the patient has had similar symptoms in the past
5. Whether the patient has a fever; and if so, the temperature

4.5 Responding to Patients' Questions

The medical office employee is qualified to answer only general, nonmedical questions. Questions which are medical in nature are referred to the physician or nurse. If the physician and nurse are unavailable, take a message so that the call can be returned later.

When a patient asks a nonmedical question, be courteous and kind. Remember, when you are talking with a patient by telephone, only the tone of your voice communicates your concern and understanding. Since the patient cannot see your facial expression, you must "put a smile" into your voice. Allow the patient plenty of time to fully explain the question and to understand your answer. Clarify the answer

Figure 4-2   Medical Message

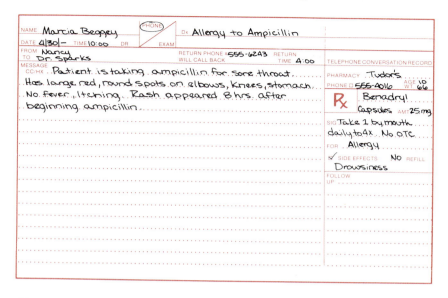

if necessary. The patient should never be made to feel that a question is unimportant or that you do not have time to be asked. Sometimes patients ask the medical office employee questions about their medical conditions or about their medication. You should tactfully refer these questions to the physician or nurse.

4.6   Handling the Doctor's Personal Calls

Almost all physicians receive some personal calls at the office. These calls may be from members of the family, from other physicians, or from the doctor's accountant, insurance representative, attorney, or stockbroker. If the doctor is not with a patient, these calls can usually be transferred. If the doctor is with a patient, personal calls are handled the same way other calls are handled, with the doctor telephoning as soon as possible. You should ask the physician which calls to transfer.

4.7   Holding

Holding is the capacity of a telephone line to hold one call while the line is being used for another call. The person on hold does not hear the other conversation. Asking a person to hold is a necessity at times; however, do not abuse nor overuse the hold capability.

Before putting a caller on hold, ask the caller's permission and give a reason. Then check back at 30-second intervals. If your business cannot be completed within one minute, ask if you can return the call. The hold function is abused when a person answers the phone by saying, "Hold, please," and immediately pushes the hold button. Another abuse of the hold function is to ask several callers to hold the line at the same time. Since it is impossible to handle three or four hold calls within one minute, take the telephone numbers and return each call as soon as possible. A caller who waits longer than a minute may think that the office employee is being rude; this may cost the practice a patient's goodwill. Always give the caller an opportunity to call back later, or offer to return the call yourself.

Proper Use of Hold

Medical Office Employee: Dr. Sparks's office. May I help you?

Caller: I'd like to make an appointment.

Medical Office Employee: I am talking to someone on another line. Would you hold the line for a moment, or may I call you back?

Improper Use of Hold

Medical Office Employee: Dr. Sparks's office. Hold, please.

4.8 Delivering Messages

Most physicians set aside special times when they return telephone calls. All routine messages should be placed on the physician's desk before these times; other messages, requiring immediate attention, should be given to the physician between examinations. Messages should not be delayed any longer than necessary since patients wait for the doctor's call.

PLACING CALLS

Wait until all patients in the office have been greeted and registered before making telephone calls. Business calls should be brief and to the point. Personal calls should be delayed until lunch or break, and they should be made out of the patients' earshot.

4.9 Outside Local Calls

Medical office employees place telephone calls for a variety of reasons. Calls may be made to patients, to other offices, to hospitals, or to suppliers. When your calls are answered, identify yourself and the medical office. If you are placing a call for the physician, identify the physician by name. If the person you are calling is not available, leave a message or explain that you will try again later.

First Call

Person Answering Phone: Good morning, American Diabetes Association.

Medical Office Employee: This is Carol Roberts from Dr. Sparks's office. The doctor will attend the American Diabetes Association luncheon tomorrow at the Berkshire Hotel.

Second Call

Person Answering Phone: Good morning, Legal Offices.

Medical Office Employee: This is Carol Roberts from Dr. Sparks's office. Dr. Sparks would like to talk about his tax credits for this year with Mrs. Goldfarb.

Person Answering Phone: I'm sorry, Mrs. Goldfarb is not in today. May I have her return the call tomorrow?

Medical Office Employee: Thank you, but we will call back tomorrow.

4.10 Making Patient Referral Appointments

When the physician wants a patient to be examined by another physician or to have medical tests done by a laboratory, the medical office employee may be asked to schedule the appointment by telephone. When making a referral call, identify yourself and the referring physician. Then give all necessary information about the patient's condition, the previous treatment, and any tests which the referring physician wishes to have performed. After the appointment has been set, give the patient a card indicating the date, time, and address of the new physician or lab.

A preprinted form can be used for keeping track of consultations and referrals. The form usually has three copies: one for the patient's folder, one for the consulting physician, and one for the patient. It lists the patient's name and age; diagnosis; the reason for the consultation or referral; date requested; referring physician's name, address, and phone number; plus comments about the case. There is space for the consulting physician's report and signature.

Maintain a list of consulting physicians with their telephone numbers since patients sometimes ask for the recommendation of a specialist.

4.11 Reminding Patients of Appointments

When appointments are made several months in advance, patients may forget the exact date and time of their scheduled visit. Therefore, some physicians ask the medical office assistant to remind patients by telephone a few days before the appointment. Reminder calls are not made for visits scheduled shortly before the appointment.

4.12 Long Distance Calls

Long distance calls may involve direct dialing or operator assistance. They may be charged to the number from which they are placed, to a credit card, to a third number, or to the individual being called (collect).

A *person-to-person call* is made when you wish to speak to a specific person. A *station-to-station call* is made when you will talk to anyone who answers the telephone. Person-to-person rates are higher than station-to-station rates, but a person-to-person call may be more economical since the charge begins only after the person you want to reach answers the phone.

Collect calls are sometimes known as "reversed calls" because the charge is reversed to the answering telephone. The individual who answers must agree to pay the charges before the operator will connect the call. A collect call can be person-to-person or station-to-station.

Collect Person-to-Person Call

Medical Office Employee: Operator, I'd like to place a collect call to Miss Alice Randall at New York Pharmaceuticals. This is Carol Roberts calling from Dr. John Sparks's office.

Operator: What number are you calling from?

Medical Office Employee: 555-4567

Operator (when phone is answered): I have a collect call for Miss Alice Randall from Carol Roberts in Dr. John Sparks's office. Will you accept the charges?

Long distance calls can be made away from the office and charged to a telephone credit card or to the office telephone. A call charged to a credit card is usually less expensive than a call charged to a third number. In either case, dial "O," the area code, and the number. The operator will then assist you in completing the call, or a recording will ask you to enter the billing code shown on your credit card.

4.13 Returning Long Distance Calls

When the individual you want to reach with a person-to-person call is out of the office, the operator leaves a message for the call to be returned. The initiator of the original call pays for the return call. To return the call, the return caller must dial the local operator ("O") and give the information shown on the call-back form. A telephone message to return a long distance call is shown in Figure 4-3.

Figure 4-3 Call-back Message Form

```
TO: Dr. Sparks                         DATE: 4/2/--
                                       TIME: 3 pm.
┌──────────────────────────────────────────────────┐
│              TELEPHONE MESSAGE                    │
└──────────────────────────────────────────────────┘
Mr. Eugene Dohoney    OF  Atec Pharmaceuticals
ADDRESS _____

┌─────────────┬───┬──────────────┬──────────────────┐
│ CALLED      │ ✓ │ WANTS TO SEE YOU │ RETURNED YOUR CALL │
├─────────────┼───┼──────────────┼──────────────────┤
│ PLEASE CALL │ ✓ │ WILL CALL AGAIN │ URGENT          │
└─────────────┴───┴──────────────┴──────────────────┘
MESSAGE  Call back operator 32
         New York City

PHONE NUMBER (212) 555-0432    TAKEN BY  HB
```

Medical Office Employee: [*Dials "0"*] Operator, I have a call back for Operator 32 in New York City.

Medical Communications

Operator 32:	This is Operator 32. What is the name and number of the person you are calling back?
Medical Office Employee:	Dr. John Sparks is returning Mr. Eugene Dohoney's call. The number is 555-0432.

4.14 Conference Calls

Long distance conversations can include several people in different cities by way of a conference call. To arrange a conference call, dial "O" and give the operator the name, area code, and telephone number of each person who will participate in the conversation. You may also ask the operator to arrange the call for a specific time. When all parties to the call are on the line, the operator contacts the originator of the call, and the conversation begins.

4.15 Directory Assistance

Most of the numbers you call are listed in the local telephone directory, the medical records, or the office telephone number file. If necessary, you can ask Directory Assistance for a number. When asking for Directory Assistance, it is important to know the correct spelling of the name you are looking for and the address; however, Directory Assistance can sometimes locate a telephone number even if you know only part of the address or possible spellings of a name.

To reach Directory Assistance for a local number, dial 1-555-1212; in some areas, local directory assistance is 411. Outside the local calling area, dial 1-area code-555-1212. Use Directory Assistance only when you cannot locate the number elsewhere; there is a charge for the service.

4.16 Telephone Number File

In order to locate telephone numbers quickly, medical offices maintain a file of phone numbers. Patient numbers are usually located in the alphabetic card file (See Section 7.26, page 122) or the medical record, while a rotary card file is maintained for business-related numbers such as the cleaning service, the electric company, and suppliers. A separate card is used for each name and telephone number (see Figure 4-4). Emergency numbers such as police, fire department, rescue squad, the doctor's personal physician, and local hospitals should be typed on a card and taped to the telephone or desk.

Figure 4-4   Rotary Telephone Number File

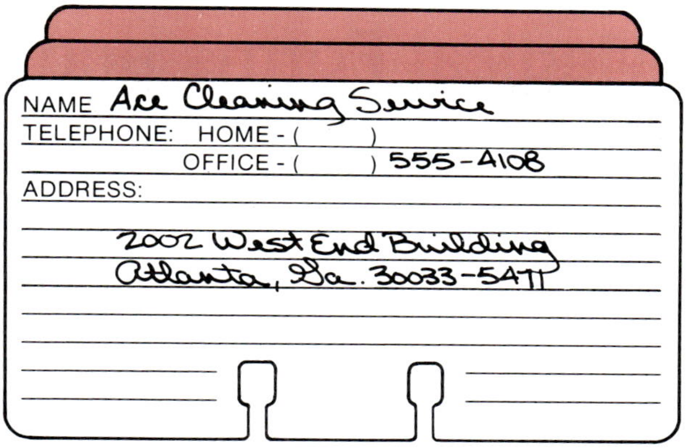

```
NAME   Ace Cleaning Service
TELEPHONE:  HOME - (     )
            OFFICE - (    ) 555-4108
ADDRESS:
       2002 West End Building
       Atlanta, Ga. 30033-5471
```

4.17   Answering Service

To be accessible at all hours, most physicians use an answering service for after-hours and weekend calls. Sometimes an automatic switching device can be used which sends calls directly to the answering service if they are not answered at the medical office. If the answering service does not switch on and off automatically, the medical office employee calls the service and tells them the time to begin answering, where the physician can be reached, and the time to stop answering. After returning to the office, the employee checks with the service for messages. Since many answering services charge according to the number of calls received and the time spent tracing the physician, you should use the service only when necessary.

Some medical offices use a recorded message to give patients a number where the physician can be reached. The message may also give regular office hours.

5

Medical Forms and Medical Reports

Medical forms and reports are found in a variety of types and styles. Some medical reports are commercially printed and include space for the physician, nurse, or other medical staff member to add information about the patient. Other reports are dictated by the physician and keyboarded by a medical office employee. Still others are prepared by health care professionals in hospitals, laboratories, or therapy centers and then sent to the medical office. All of these reports are stored in the medical records. The descriptions and illustrations which follow are typical of some of the medical reports developed for a general or internal medical practice. For other specialties, customized reports are available from medical office supply firms.

PATIENT-COMPLETED FORMS

5.1 Patient Information Form

The *patient information form* shown in Figure 5-1 is completed by the patient immediately upon arrival at the medical office for the initial visit. Information requested on the form includes personal information about the patient; the name, address, and telephone number of the person responsible for payment (the guarantor); the names, addresses, and policy numbers for all health insurance companies with whom the patient has coverage; the employer's name and address; and the name of the referring physician. The patient information form is the basis for creating the patient file and for filing health insurance claims.

5.2 Patient Health Questionnaire

Physicians need background health information about patients in order to provide the best treatment. The *patient questionnaire* is designed for this purpose. This questionnaire asks about the patient's

Chapter 5—Medical Forms and Reports 61

Figure 5-1 Patient Information Form

PATIENT INFORMATION

Please Print Clearly   DATE SEPT. 9, 19--

NAME NATHAN LEE   AGE 45   SEX M

_____12/7/41_____ ☐ SINGLE   ☐ MARRIED   ☐ WIDOWED   ☒ DIVORCED
BIRTH DATE

ADDRESS 1071 FULTON DR.

CITY ATLANTA   STATE GEORGIA   ZIP 30312-1768

PHONE 555-0542   OCCUPATION SALES REPRESENTATIVE

EMPLOYED BY FEZCO, INC.

CITY ATLANTA   STATE GEORGIA   ZIP 30316-9502

SPOUSE'S NAME NA

EMPLOYED BY NA

CITY NA   STATE NA   ZIP NA

PHONE NA   OCCUPATION NA

REFERRED BY DR. ABNER DOWARKSIK

MEDICAL INSURANCE? ☒ YES ☐ NO   SURGICAL? ☒ YES ☐ NO

MEDICAL INSURANCE GROUP NO. GA66951   CERTIFICATE NO. 475

COMPANY STONE MOUNTAIN GENERAL

SURGICAL INSURANCE GROUP NO. 1765   CERTIFICATE NO. 818

COMPANY UNITED SURGICAL PLAN

NAME NATHAN LEE
(PERSON RESPONSIBLE FOR PAYMENT)

ADDRESS 1071 FULTON DR.

CITY ATLANTA   STATE GEORGIA   ZIP 30312-1768

family health history, the patient's personal health and surgical history, the patient's allergies, and X rays that the patient has undergone. In addition, the questionnaire seeks information about the patient's bodily systems, immunizations, and personal habits.

Some physicians prefer that the patient complete the questionnaire while other physicans feel that the questionnaire is more thoroughly completed when a medical office employee questions the patient and completes the form. Many questionnaires provide space for background health information and leave room for the doctor's notes on subsequent visits. Customized questionnaires designed for each specialty are available from medical office supply firms. A patient health questionnaire is shown in Figure 5-2.

PHYSICIAN-COMPLETED FORMS

5.3 Case History

The patient's *case history* is dictated by the physician and transcribed by a medical office employee after the initial visit. The case history describes (1) the patient's complaint or physical problem, (2) results of the physical examination, (3) results of lab tests, (4) the physician's diagnosis, (5) the prescribed treatment for the physical problem, (6) remarks the physician thinks are pertinent to the patient's case, (7) a family history, and (8) a personal history. The case history is stored in the patient's medical record for reference. A case history is shown in Figure 5-3, page 64.

5.4 Physical Examination Form

As the physician examines the patient, the results are recorded on a *physical examination form*. This form is used as a reference for changing physical conditions and is stored with the case history in the medical record. A physical examination form is shown in Figure 5-4, page 64.

5.5 Doctor's Notes

Doctor's notes, or *progress notes,* are added to the medical record each time the patient is treated. After the person is examined, the physician or nurse records notes about the condition, diagnosis, and treatment in chronological order on the patient health questionnaire or on a blank, standard-sized sheet of paper. Prescriptions and telephone consultations are also recorded in chronological order. All notes are initialed by the person who writes them. Refer to Figure 5-5, page 65, for an illustration of doctor's notes.

Chapter 5—Medical Forms and Reports

Figure 5-2 Patient Health Questionnaire

PATIENT'S NAME Marvin Connelly
ADDRESS 610 Shady Lane   INSURANCE Metropolitan   DATE 3/4/--
TEL NO 242-4261   REFERRED BY John Lazarus   OCCUPATION Carpenter   AGE 29   SEX M   S M W D

FAMILY HISTORY: FATHER Deceased   MOTHER Healthy   BROTHERS 1   SISTERS 2
CANCER _____ TUBERCULOSIS _____ INSANITY _____ DIABETES Father   HEART DISEASE _____ RHEUMATISM _____
GOUT _____ GOITER _____ OBESITY Father   NEPHRITIS _____ EPILEPSY _____ OTHER _____
PAST HISTORY: DIPHTHERIA _____ MEASLES ✓   MUMPS ✓   SCARLET FEVER _____ SMALL POX _____ INFANTILE PARALYSIS _____
TYPHOID _____ PNEUMONIA _____ INFECTIONS _____ GONORRHEA _____ SYPHILIS _____ TONSILLITIS ✓   OPERATIONS None
MENSTRUAL: ONSET _____ PERIODICITY _____ TYPE _____ DURATION _____ PAIN _____ L M P _____
MARITAL: MISCARRIAGES _____ ABORTIONS _____ CHILDREN _____ STERILITY _____
HABITS: ALCOHOL Moderate   TOBACCO N/A   DRUGS N/A   COFFEE 2 cups/day   MEALS heavy   WATER 3 cups/day
SLEEP 7 hrs/night   BOWEL MOVEMENTS Regular   EXERCISE Light   AMUSEMENTS Bowling
PRESENT AILMENT Back pain, especially painful when lying down. Pain started about 1 week ago in lower back — has moved upward
PHYSICAL EXAMINATION: TEMP. 99.2   PULSE 100   RESP 16   B P 130/90   HEIGHT 6'1"   WEIGHT 195
SKIN Normal   MUCOUS MEMBRANE Normal   EYES Normal Limits   EARS no redness or drainage   NOSE Normal   MOUTH Normal
NECK Supple   CHEST Normal   LUNGS Bilateral breath sounds   HEART Normal tones   ABDOMEN Soft   RECTUM Normal
VAGINA _____ GENITALS _____ EXTREMITIES _____ OTHER _____
LABORATORY FINDINGS: Xray normal
DIAGNOSIS: Back strain
TREATMENT: Heat, rest
REMARKS: _____

| DATE | | | SUBSEQUENT VISITS AND FINDINGS | CASE NO. |
MO.	DAY	YR.		
12	20	--	Laceration of third finger left hand p.i.p. joint. Good movement, no tendon damage. 3, 5-0 prolene sutures	

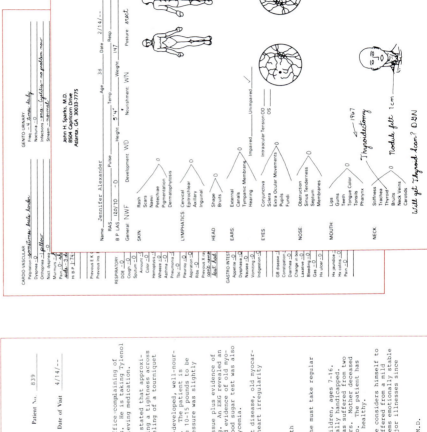

Figure 5-3 Case History

Figure 5-4 Physical Examination Form

Figure 5-5 Doctor's Notes

5	18	--	URI – stuffy nose, sore throat, sleeplessness Ampicillin #20 t.i.d. till gone
8	10	--	Warts on hand – removed with liquid nitrogen. Return in 1 week for reevaluation.

LABORATORY REPORTS

A wide variety of laboratory tests are administered to identify medical problems. Some minor laboratory tests are performed in the office, while an outside lab is used for major tests. Reports of the results, called *lab reports,* are stored in the medical record. Several common laboratory tests and reporting forms are described in the following section.

5.6 Laboratory Requests

When a patient requires laboratory tests, a form is completed listing the tests to be administered and the name of the attending physician. A laboratory request is shown in Figure 5-6, page 66.

5.7 Urinalysis

One of the first laboratory tests administered to many patients is an examination of the urine. From urine tests, a physician can determine if infection is present in the body, if a woman is pregnant, if diabetes mellitus is indicated, or if a variety of other conditions exist. A urinalysis report is shown in Figure 5-7, page 66.

Figure 5-6 Laboratory Request

```
                    LABORATORY REQUEST

    John H. Sparks, M.D.                       555-0078
    8504 Capricorn Drive
    Atlanta, GA  30033-7775

    Date  4/16/--

    To  Rachel Morgan
        Briarcliff Labs
    Re  Susanne Snoffer

    Please perform the following tests:
    ☐ Culture of _____
    ☐ C S F for _____
    ☐ Feces for _____
    ☐ E K G _____
    ☐ B M R _____
    ☐ Pregnancy _____
    ☒ Urinalysis _____
    ☐ H P N _____
    ☒ Blood Sugar _____
    ☐ R H Factor & Blood Type _____
    ☐ SED Rate _____
    ☒ W B C & Diff _____
    ☐ R B C & H G D _____
    ☐ Other _____


                    John H. Sparks, M.D.
                         Signature
```

Figure 5-7 Urinalysis Report

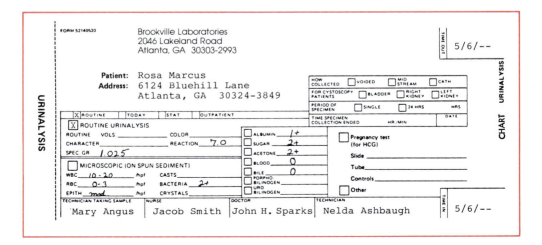

5.8 Electrocardiogram

An *electrocardiogram* is a graphic illustration of the activity of the heart. It is used by physicians to diagnose and treat heart conditions. Electrocardiograms, taken at time intervals such as every six months or once a year, are compared to determine whether any change has taken place in the heart's activity. The results are stored with other diagnostic tests in the medical record. An electrocardiogram report showing a cardiologist's notes is shown in Figure 5-8.

Figure 5-8 Electrocardiogram Report

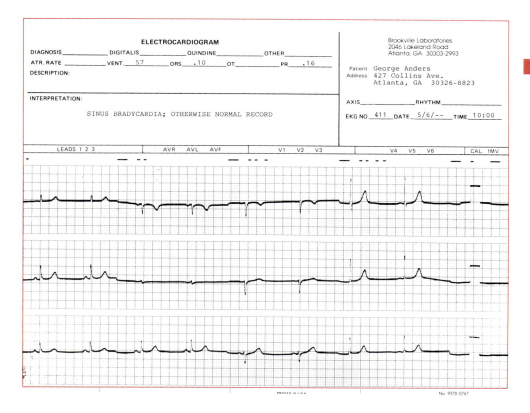

5.9 Blood Tests

Blood tests can reveal whether infection is present in the body, whether urea is present in the blood, whether glucose (sugar) is concentrated in the blood, and many other conditions. Many forms exist for reporting the results of blood tests. A blood test reporting form is shown in Figure 5-9, page 68.

Figure 5-9 Blood Test Reporting Form

5.10 Radiology Reports

Radiology is commonly associated with X rays. However, in addition to X rays, radiologists perform other diagnostic procedures such as CAT scans and ultrasound examinations. An *X ray* is a picture of an internal body part. By analyzing or *reading* an X ray, a radiologist can see if anything is medically unusual about the body part. After the radiologist reads the X ray, a formal report is sent to the primary care physican. X rays are usually too large to store in the medical record, so they are stored in large envelopes in a separate location. Only the radiologist's report is stored in the medical record. A radiologist's report of a patient's thyroid scan is shown in Figure 5-10.

5.11 Pathology Reports

Pathology is the branch of medicine which studies body tissue. *Cytopathology* is a branch of pathology concerned with the study of body cells to identify medical conditions. Cells are often removed from a patient's body and sent to a pathology lab for testing to determine whether disease is present. The Pap smear is an example of a commonly performed cytopathology test. A typical reporting form from a cytopathology laboratory is shown in Figure 5-11.

5.12 Shingling Reports

Since laboratory reports are often small and of irregular size, they can be easily lost. Consequently, *shingling*—a method of attaching reports to a standard-sized sheet of paper—is used in many offices.

Chapter 5—Medical Forms and Reports 69

Figure 5-10 Radiology Report

```
                                            Patient's Name  Jennifer Alexander
                                            Hosp No
             DEPARTMENT OF RADIOLOGY        Room No
             NUCLEAR MEDICINE REPORT        Ref Physician

                                    Nuclear                Pregnant
 Date  3/15/--                      Medicine No  005375
 Examination               Isotopic Compound    Dose       Ancillary Studies
   Thyroid Scan
   I 131 Uptake              Sodium I 131
```

The patient has had a thyroidectomy for hyperthyroidism. A 24-hour radioactive iodine uptake is .08% reflecting the surgical removal of the thyroid. A small area of functioning thyroid tissue is seen to the right of the midline probably in the region of the upper pole of the thyroid. There is no evidence of activity in the lower left midline neck in the region of the palpable nodule.

Dr. Sabina Gwyn

NUCLEAR MEDICINE REPORT

Figure 5-11 Cytopathology Report

```
                              METROPOLITAN HOSPITAL  CYTOLOGY      C— 19-- 0000
                              ATLANTA, GA
 Brookville Laboratories      ☒ GENITAL              ☐ NON GENITAL
 2046 Lakeland Road
 Atlanta, GA  30303-2993      ☒ CERVICAL           ☐ SPUTUM      ☐ GASTRIC
                              ☐ VAGINAL            ☐ URINE       ☐ SMALL INT
 Patient:  Rosa Marcus   Age: 45   ☐ MATURITY INDEX  ☐ BREAST   ☐ LARGE INT
 Address  6124 Bluehill Lane                        ☐ PLEURAL    ☐ OTHER
          Atlanta, GA  30324-3849                   ☐ PERITONEAL
                              ☐ LAB USE ONLY        ☐ BRON WASH
 CLINICAL INFORMATION:        PREVIOUS SMEARS ____ 19__  ☐ BRON BRUSH
 LAST MENSTRUAL PERIOD: 6/3/--  DIAGNOSIS  NEGATIVE      ☐ CSF
                              PREGNANT  YES ☐  NO ☒     ☐ ESOPH
                              YEARS POSTMENOPAUSAL
 CONSULTATION REPORT:    REMARKS:                   Date: 6/24/--
 ☐ UNSATISFACTORY    ☐ POSITIVE
 ☒ NEGATIVE          ☐ IN SITU
 ☐ NO ENDOCERVICALS  ☐ INVASIVE
 ☐ ATYPICAL BENIGN   ☐ OTHER
 ☐ DYSPLASIA
                              Nelda Ashbaugh        John H. Sparks M.D.
                                CYTOTECHNOLOGIST       PATHOLOGIST
```

CHART COPY

This method allows related reports, such as blood test results, to be secured together on a standard-sized sheet of paper. The report with the earliest date is attached to the bottom of the sheet and the report with the second earliest date is attached to the top of the first, approximately one-half inch above the bottom of the first report. This procedure continues, with succeeding reports being attached closer to the top of the sheet. Shingled lab reports are shown in Figure 5-12. If laboratory reports are not shingled, they should be taped to a blank sheet of paper before being stored in the medical record.

Figure 5-12 Shingled Lab Reports

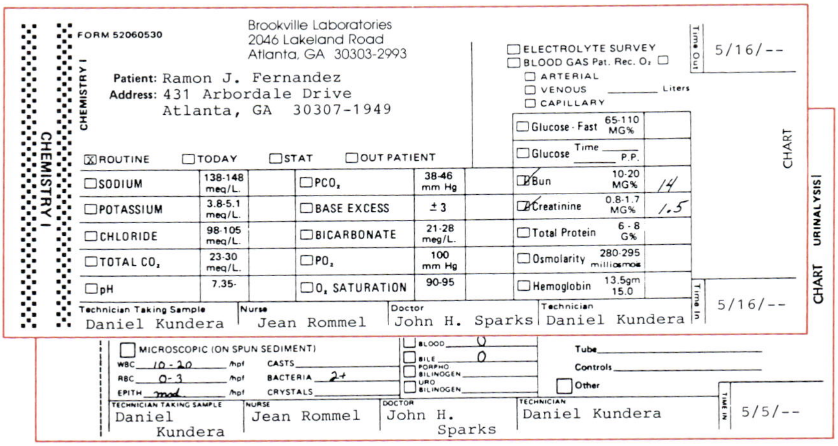
FORM 52060530
Brookville Laboratories
2046 Lakeland Road
Atlanta, GA 30303-2993
CHEMISTRY I
Patient: Ramon J. Fernandez
Address: 431 Arbordale Drive
Atlanta, GA 30307-1949
ELECTROLYTE SURVEY
BLOOD GAS Pat. Rec. O₂
ARTERIAL
VENOUS ______ Liters
CAPILLARY
Time Out 5/16/--

[X] ROUTINE TODAY STAT OUT PATIENT

SODIUM	138-148 meq/L.	PCO₂	38-46 mm Hg	Glucose - Fast	65-110 MG%
POTASSIUM	3.8-5.1 meq/L.	BASE EXCESS	± 3	Glucose Time ____ P.P.	
CHLORIDE	98-105 meq/L.	BICARBONATE	21-28 meq/L.	Bun	10-20 MG% 14
TOTAL CO₂	23-30 meq/L.	PO₂	100 mm Hg	Creatinine	0.8-1.7 MG% 1.5
pH	7.35-	O₂ SATURATION	90-95	Total Protein	6-8 G%
				Osmolarity	280-295 milliosmos
				Hemoglobin	13.5gm 15.0

Technician Taking Sample: Daniel Kundera Nurse: Jean Rommel Doctor: John H. Sparks Technician: Daniel Kundera Time In 5/16/--

CHART CHART URINALYSIS I

MICROSCOPIC (ON SPUN SEDIMENT)
WBC 10-20 /hpf CASTS
RBC 0-3 /hpf BACTERIA 2+
EPITH mod /hpf CRYSTALS
BLOOD 0
BILE 0
PORPHO BILINOGEN
URO BILINOGEN
Tube
Controls
Other
Technician Taking Sample: Daniel Kundera Nurse: Jean Rommel Doctor: John H. Sparks Technician: Daniel Kundera Time In 5/5/--

HOSPITAL REPORTS

During the time a patient is hospitalized, several reports are generated at the hospital. The admitting summary and the discharge summary are dictated by the admitting physician, and additional reports such as laboratory reports, pathology reports, and consulting reports are generated by other health care professionals. Reports developed in the hospital are included in the hospital record; the admitting history and discharge summary also are sent to the admitting physician's office for inclusion in the patient's medical record. Three major reports dictated by physicians are described below.

5.13 Admitting History

The admitting history is dictated by the admitting physician after the patient enters the hospital. It includes information about the patient's complaint, the results of the physician's examination, the diagnosis, the prescribed treatment, a personal health history, and a family health history. The hospital admitting history is similar to the case history described in Section 5.3.

5.14 Discharge Summary

The discharge summary is dictated by the admitting physician at the time the patient is discharged from the hospital. The discharge summary includes (1) the dates of admission and discharge; (2) the admission diagnosis or the reason for hospitalization; (3) the discharge diagnosis or the findings; (4) operations and procedures; (5) condensed history and physical; (6) laboratory, pathology, and X ray results; (7) the hospital course of treatment; (8) prescriptions, medications, and instructions; and (9) the disposition of the case. A patient's hospital records are not considered complete until the discharge summary is included. A discharge summary is illustrated in Figure 5-13.

Figure 5-13 Discharge Summary

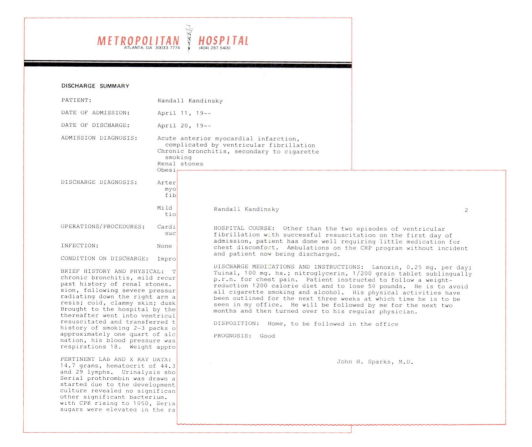

5.15 Consultation Report

Primary care physicians frequently ask other physicians to consult on their hospitalization cases. The consulting physician prepares a consultation report which is sent to the primary care physician for review and for inclusion in the medical record. An illustration of a consultation report is shown in Figure 5-14.

Figure 5-14 Consultation Report

Lucas Johnson, M.D., Inc.   953 Peachtree Ct.   Atlanta, GA 30319-1579

```
DATE OF REQUEST:              6/3/--
CONSULTATION WITH:            Dr. Josefina Nieves
FROM:                         Dr. Lucas Johnson
OPINION REQUESTED IN REGARD TO: George B. Anders.  Chronic con-
                              gestive heart failure, secondary
                              to cardiomyopathy.  Cardiac
                              arrest this afternoon.  Conges-
                              tive heart failure with persis-
                              tent right pleural effusion.
DATE OF CONSULTATION:         6/4/--
FINDINGS:
```

failure in 1...
an outpatient...
progressed, a...
congestive he...
progressive.
at Johns Hop...
congestive ca...
coronary arte...
moderate mit...
dilatation.
origin, due t...
beverage. He...
a hemorrhoid...
cholecystitis
also known be...
and depressi...
Because the ...
ferred via p...
5/26/84. He...
when he was ...
episodes of ...
intermittent
adequately e...
these were du...
mented by an...
episode in A...
tubular necr...
ple thoracent...
any etiology
ure.

On physical ...
arrest, the p...
emaciated, w...
age. The bl...
can be palpa...

CONSULTATION REPORT

CONTINUED - PAGE TWO

When the patient was able to breathe spontaneously, the endo-tracheal tube was removed. The abdomen was extremely distended, and accordingly a nasogastric tube was passed into the stomach, and the abdomen decompressed. Central venous pressure apparatus was inserted, via the percutaneous technique into the right subclavian vein and guided into the mid-right atrium. This was performed after the patient had been transferred to the Coronary Care Unit. The central venous pressure was 38 cm. of water. Levophed was begun, but the patient's blood pressure was still not audible, although he was becoming more alert, in regards to his sensorium. He moved all extremities, and Demerol, intra-venously, was given because of dyspnea and agitation. The stat chest X ray revealed the continued presence of a marked right pleural effusion, and accordingly thoracenteses at 3-levels was performed, revealing presumably loculated fluid of about a total of 200 cc. This was a deep orange and somewhat serosanguineous. It was clear, however. Arterial blood gases and laboratory studies were sent for appropriate analyses.

IMPRESSION: Congestive cardiomyopathy with
                              myocardial irritability and
marked congestive heart failure, with right pleural effusion. The X ray configuration of the heart suggests a pericardial effusion, as well, but most likely this just reflects the chronic congestive changes and dilatation.
                              Cardiac arrest, presumably
secondary to a recurrent episode of ventricular tachycardia. Pulmonary emboli cannot be excluded.

PLANS: As soon as the blood work is
                              returned, the patient will be
diuresed following his central venous pressure closely. Acute tubular necrosis will be looked for, and treated appropriately. His situation is very grave, and the seriousness was again explained to the family.
                              Other diagnoses unchanged, as
listed in the history of present illness.

6/10/-- pk

MEDICAL RECORD PROCEDURES

5.16 Problem-Oriented Medical Record

A commonly used method of recording information is called the *problem-oriented medical record (POMR)*. In a medical office which uses this method, the patient's complaints are seen as a series of problems. The problems are identified from the initial case history, the physical examination, and the results of diagnostic tests and procedures. Each problem is given a number. This number is used when referring to treatments and procedures performed to correct the problem. Each time the patient returns for treatment of a recurring problem, the reference number for the problem is written before the doctor's notes about the visit. If more than one problem is addressed, the number of each problem is listed, along with the treatment and procedures. When a patient describes a new complaint, the complaint is added to the problem list and given a number. The problem list is stored in a prominent location in the medical record so anyone reviewing the record can locate it. Many offices staple the list to the left side of the folder.

The doctor's notes, or progress notes, for a POMR follow an established formula called SOAP. After the problem is identified and numbered, the doctor's notes are organized using the initials *S-O-A-P:*

S. Subjective—information based on the patient's feelings (feels bad, no energy, headaches). The subjective analysis is written in the patient's own words and includes the chief complaint.
O. Objective—information based on the results of diagnostic tests and procedures. These are symptoms that can be seen or proved (bruises, high blood pressure, fever).
A. Assessment—diagnosis of the problem based on subjective and objective data.
P. Plan—manner in which problem will be managed. The plan usually consists of three parts: (1) medical management, including medication, diet, and therapy; (2) diagnostic follow-up, including X rays and additional lab tests; and (3) patient education, including reinforcement of the physician's instructions by the medical office employee.

A problem-oriented medical record is shown in Figure 5-15.

5.17 Source-Oriented Medical Record

In a *source-oriented medical record (SOMR),* similar forms and reports are stored together. For example, all laboratory reports are stored in one section, while all consultation reports are stored in another. When a report is needed, all of the reports of that category must be

Figure 5-15 Problem-Oriented Medical Record

PROGRESS NOTES

Patient's Name *Michael Brandy*   Page *1*

Date	Problem Number	S-O-A-P
		S: Subjective
		O: Objective
		A: Assessment
		P: Plan
9/14/--	1	S: Stuffy nose, sore throat, sleeplessness
		O: Fever 101°, throat red
		A: URI
		P: Ampicillin #20, t.i.d. till gone; plenty of rest, plenty of fluids, well-balanced diet.

reviewed in order to determine which relates to the present illness. All urinalysis reports, for example, may have to be reviewed to determine which relates to a patient's current bladder problem. All X ray reports may have to be reviewed to determine which relates to a current lung ailment.

5.18 Chronological or Integrated Record

In a *chronological* or *integrated record*, all reports for one illness are stored in chronological order. For example, the doctor's notes for an illness are stored with the X ray reports and the laboratory reports for the same illness. The chronological method was traditionally used to store materials in the medical record until the POMR was instituted at major medical schools.

5.19 Confidentiality

Confidentiality of medical records is a major concern for medical offices. In addition to the ethics of confidentiality, physicians are legally bound to keep all patient materials confidential. A physician can be prosecuted if confidential information is released by the medical office staff (see Section 2.5).

MISCELLANEOUS MEDICAL FORMS

A variety of medical forms which aid in patient care do not fall into well-defined categories. Several of these forms are described below.

5.20 Introduction of Patient

When patients are referred to a consulting physician, a note or letter of referral is sent to the new physician. A patient referral form is shown in Figure 5-16, page 76.

5.21 Certification of Illness or Health by Physician

Students and employees often need a doctor's note before they can be excused from a school or work activity. A notarized certification of illness sometimes becomes a part of the legal record in a court case. A certificate of health is sometimes necessary for the same reasons.

A certification of illness is shown in Figure 5-17. A certification of health is shown in Figure 5-18. (see page 76)

76 Medical Communications

Figure 5-16 Patient Referral Form

```
John H. Sparks, M.D.                           555-0078
8504 Capricorn Dr.
Atlanta, GA  30033-7775           Date 2/10/--

To  Sandra Duncan, M.D.
    8024 Limelight Drive
    Atlanta, GA  30304-7773

This will present my patient,
Virginia Brismer
for the following: ☒ Diagnosis
                   ☐ Treatment
☒ Case history is enclosed
                                     Remarks
Review for possible
hyperthyroidism.


              John H. Sparks, M.D.
                   Signature
```

Figure 5-17 Certification of Illness

```
John H. Sparks, M.D.                           555-0078
8504 Capricorn Dr.
Atlanta, GA  30033-7775

              Date 2/17/--

This will certify that
Virginia Brismer
is under my care for the following:
hyperthyroidism


              John H. Sparks, M.D.
                   Signature
```

Figure 5-18 Certification of Health

```
          CERTIFICATE OF HEALTH

John H. Sparks, M.D.                           555-0078
8504 Capricorn Dr.
Atlanta, GA  30033-7775

              Date 3/4/--

This will certify that
Lucinda Sars
is free of any contagious or infectious disease and has
my permission to attend school.


              John H. Sparks, M.D.
                   Signature
```

Chapter 5—Medical Forms and Reports   **77**

5.22   Disability Certificate

Physicians are sometimes asked to certify a patient's disability for an employer or a school. A disability certificate is shown in Figure 5-19, page 78.

5.23   Authorization for Records Release

The patient's signed permission is necessary before information about the patient can be released to anyone, including the insurance company. For minors, the parent or guardian's signature is needed. An authorization to release information is shown in Figure 5-20, page 78.

5.24   Authority to Operate

Before a physician is allowed to operate at a hospital, the hospital requires a signed *authority to operate*. The form must be signed by the patient or the patient's family member. An authority to operate form is shown in Figure 5-21, page 78.

PROCEDURE FOR TYPING MEDICAL REPORTS

5.25   Margins and Spacing

When a medical report is typed on a ruled form, begin the left margin at the far left edge of the line. End the right margin at the far right edge of the line. When a medical report is typed on plain paper, use a standard 60-space line and leave a one-inch top and bottom margin. Use single spacing for long reports and double spacing for short reports.

5.26   Tables

When a table is a part of a medical report, leave equal space between all columns. If possible, space the columns so you can use the standard tabs on your word processor. Center the headings over each column. With modern office equipment, it is no longer necesssary to count characters and divide in order to determine column spacing. Visually attractive spacing is usually adequate.

Figure 5-19 Disability Certificate

DISABILITY CERTIFICATE 555-0078

John H. Sparks, M.D.
8504 Capricorn Dr.
Atlanta, GA 30033-7775

Date: 6/10/--

This will certify that Anson Lobock

has been under my care and was
☐ Totally incapacitated
☑ Partially incapacitated

From 5/14/-- to 6/10/--

Remarks: Fracture of lower tibia

John H. Sparks, M.D.
Signature

Figure 5-20 Authorization to Release Information

RECORDS RELEASE AUTHORIZATION

TO: JOHN H. SPARKS, M.D.
8504 CAPRICORN DR.
ATLANTA, GA 30033-7775

I authorize and request you to release to:
TALL PINES CLINIC
1757 CLIFTON ROAD
ATLANTA, GA 30033-9950

the complete history and record of my illness and/or treatment during the period

from 5/14/-- to 6/10/--
Name: ANSON LOBOCK
Date: 6/12/--

Anson Lobock
Signature (if relative, state relationship)

Jennifer Gale
Witness

Figure 5-21 Authority to Operate Form

AUTHORITY TO OPERATE   Date 3/4/--

I, Jason Wheeler
     patient's name

of 3462 Stone Mountain Road
   Decatur, GA 30033-1117

hereby grant authority to

John H. Sparks, M.D.
8504 Capricorn Dr.
Atlanta, GA 30033-7775

and/or to the doctor(s) in charge of the care of the patient whose name appears above, to administer any treatment or to administer such anesthetics, and to perform such operations as may be deemed necessary or advisable in the diagnosis and treatment of this patient.

Jason Wheeler
Signature of patient or nearest relative

Relationship _Patient_

Authorization to be signed by patient, or if patient is incompetent or a minor, the nearest relative.

6

Medical Correspondence

INCOMING MAIL

The task of opening and preparing the daily mail is an important responsibility. Depending on the size of your medical office, you may receive the mail directly from the postal carrier at your desk or obtain the mail for your department from the mailroom of your medical facility.

6.1   Opening the Mail

Before you open the mail, separate it into categories such as business correspondence, medical publications, and advertising. Business correspondence, which includes medical laboratory reports, should be opened first. Use a letter opener to make the job easier and to preserve the mailing envelopes. Confidential mail, or any mail marked *personal*, should not be opened. This mail should be given directly to the addressee as soon as possible.

6.2   Review the Mail and Enclosures

As you open each piece of mail, quickly scan all letters and note any enclosures mentioned. Make certain the enclosures were actually sent with the letter. If they are missing, attach a small note or make a pencil notation on the letter indicating that an enclosure is missing. Then call the office that sent the letter and ask that the enclosure be sent as soon as possible. Write the date, the name of the person you spoke to, and the telephone number you called on the note you attach to the letter.

6.3   Save the Return Address

As you review the mail and all enclosures, look to see if the return address of the sender is included on the inside correspondence before discarding the envelope. If not, save the envelope as a record of the return address. If the return address is shown on the letter, you can discard the envelope unless your office has a policy of keeping envelopes. Sometimes offices keep envelopes to have the date of the postmark—the mark the Postal Service uses to cancel the stamp.

6.4 Date the Mail

Most offices will have a date stamp to use with the mail. The stamp may include office or department information and even the time. It is important to know when mail is received in order to monitor office efficiency, especially how quickly patient inquiries are answered. Most medical offices prefer that the date be stamped on the back, or in a specific location on the front of the mail. Check with your supervisor to determine office preference. Never stamp the date over typed information.

On pictures or glossy brochures where the date stamp might rub off, you can put the date stamp on a small piece of paper and attach that to the item. Check the doctor's preference for dating medical reference materials, magazines, and advertisements.

6.5 Sort the Mail

If you sort the mail for many individuals or several departments, you may have to sort the mail by individual or department. Next sort the opened mail according to the following categories:

- Category I: Urgent or emergency mail
- Category II: Unopened personal or confidential mail
- Category III: Routine correspondence
- Category IV: Bills or invoices
- Category V: Medical research magazines or journals
- Category VI: Other magazines, newspapers
- Category VII: Advertisements

After you become familiar with the mail procedures, you will find that you can sort while you open and date the mail.

6.6 Attach Related Files

Another useful mail-handling procedure is to retrieve files related to the mail and attach them to the mail. The doctor or technician can then refer to the file and respond to the mail quickly. Check with your supervisor for your office's procedure.

Chapter 6—Medical Correspondence 81

6.7 Delivering the Mail

The mail should be opened, sorted, and delivered as soon as it is received. Always place opened mail in a folder to maintain confidentiality. If a large volume of mail is received, it is a good idea to have separate folders for the various mail categories. Ask the doctor where to put the opened mail. The location the doctor suggests should be used consistently.

If the mail is to be placed in the doctor's office, do not take it in while the doctor is with a patient or on the telephone. Wait until the doctor is free before taking in the mail.

Bills and invoices may be directed to the office manager or bookkeeper, and general magazines should be placed in the reception area for patients. When you are first assigned the task of opening the mail, find out how the mail should be directed in your office. Ask questions, or consult the office procedures manual.

6.8 Mail Logs

Mail logs may be maintained for registered or certified mail, insured mail, special delivery mail, mail including payments, or legal correspondence. Depending on the regulations to be followed, your office may require that some mail be logged.

Figure 6-1 Sample Mail Log Entries

Today's Date	Article	From	Date Sent	Date Received	Referred	
					To	Date
8/14	Registered letter	Dr. Avery	8/11	8/14	Dr. Sparks	8/14
8/15	X rays/ Anne Hill	Dr. Bregner	8/14	8/14	Dr. Buxton	8/15
8/16	EKG/ Nathan Lee	Dr. Avery	8/15	8/16	Dr. Sparks	8/16

PREPARING THE DOCTOR'S CORRESPONDENCE

The appearance of the correspondence leaving your office is very important. How your letter looks to the recipient—the way it is centered on the page, how neatly the errors are corrected, the grammar and punctuation, and the skill with which your message is conveyed—will create an immediate mental impression of your medical office. From the initial preparation to the final review before mailing, your responsibility in preparing medical correspondence is to make certain that you have created the best possible impression. While grammar and punctuation guidelines are discussed in other sections of this manual, this chapter will review the basic guidelines for typing business letters.

6.9 Medical Office Letterhead

Medical office letterhead is used for letters sent outside of the medical office. This letterhead is printed on good quality bond paper and contains essential information such as the name, address, and telephone number(s) of the medical organization, and a listing of doctors in the office or department. Since both the printing and the quality of paper make letterhead expensive, you should use it carefully.

Several different letterheads may be used within the same medical office. For example, in a small medical partnership each doctor may have an individual letterhead as well as the letterhead representing the medical office. In a larger medical organization, such as a hospital, the same basic letterhead might be used throughout the organization, with a variety of listings added for specific departments or individuals. The printed letterhead takes up 1½ to 2 inches at the top of the page.

Note from the examples shown below that the two-letter state abbreviations and ZIP Codes are used in the letterhead.

Figure 6-2 Medical Office Letterhead

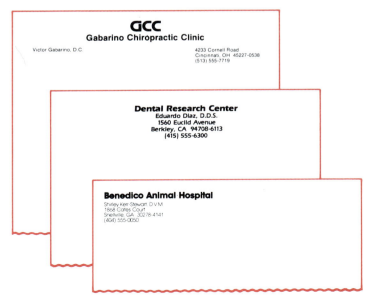

Chapter 6—Medical Correspondence   83

6.10 Letter Margins

Just as you would center a picture within a picture frame for attractive placement, so should you center the text of a letter within the margins of the page. Once you have had practice judging margins, you will find that you can quickly visualize where to place a letter. Until you have perfected this technique, however, a few guidelines will be helpful.

Most typewriters use one of two sizes of type—pica or elite. Pica type is larger and fits 10 letters into an inch. Elite type is smaller and fits 12 letters into an inch. With both styles, 6 lines are typed in 1 vertical inch.

Figure 6-3 Horizontal and Vertical Measures

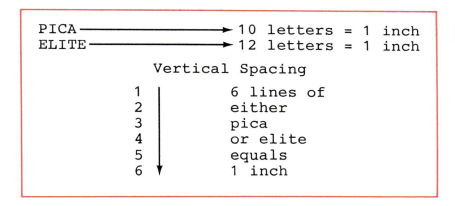

One of the first steps in determining the most attractive margins to use for business letters is to estimate what size your letter will be. Generally, letters fall into four size categories:

Table 6-1
Letter Margins

	Five-Stroke Words in Letter Body	Width of Margins	**Spaces in Margins Pica/Elite**
Small	Up to 125	2"	20 // 24
Medium	126 - 225	1 1/2"	15 // 18
Large	226 - 325	1"	10 // 12
Two Page	326 +	1"	10 // 12

While the bottom margin of your letter will vary depending on total letter length, always leave a bottom margin of at least 6 blank lines (1 inch).

If you use word processing in your medical office, you will use the same letter style and side margins in all medical correspondence.

6.11 Medical Office Letter Styles

Before you begin typing a letter, you must choose which medical office letter style to use. The horizontal placement of the dateline and other letter parts depends on the letter style.

- **Block.** All lines begin at the left margin. See Figure 6-4.

- **Modified Block with Block Paragraphs.** All lines begin at the left margin except date, complimentary close, and signature lines, which begin at the center of the page. See Figure 6-5.

- **Modified Block with Indented Paragraphs.** Identical to the modified block style mentioned above, except that all paragraphs are indented five spaces. Also, the subject line may be centered or indented five spaces to match the paragraphs. See Figure 6-6, page 86.

6.12 Personal Business Letter

If you are typing a personal business letter, use your home address as a letterhead (Figure 6-7, page 86). All other guidelines for business letter preparation should then be followed.

6.13 Punctuation Styles

Two basic punctuation styles are used in medical offices today. *Mixed punctuation* is used most frequently. It requires a colon after the salutation and a comma after the complimentary close. *Open punctuation* means that no punctuation is used after the salutation or the complimentary close.

6.14 Date

The date is an important and required part of medical correspondence. It indicates to the reader when the letter was written. To determine the vertical placement of the date, choose one of the two methods of dateline placement. The style of letterhead used in your medical office should be considered in deciding where the date looks best.

Floating Dateline. The most common method of placing the date on medical correspondence involves the floating dateline—a dateline that "floats" or moves in vertical position according to the letter size. The

Chapter 6—Medical Correspondence 85

Figure 6-4 Block Letter Style

DE ZAYAS MEDICAL OFFICE SUPPLY COMPANY
71066 Carl Street
Lauderdale, MN 55113 1066

April 29, 19--

SPECIAL DELIVERY

Patrick W. Gettings, M.D.
Austin Medical Research Center
2704 San Pedro
Austin, TX 78705-1176

Dear Dr. Gettings:

It is a pleasure to enclose a copy of our new catalog of medical office supplies. You will be pleased to see that we have noted the suggestions of countless medical offices such as yours and included 50 new items in this edition.

A 10 percent discount will be available for all orders accompanied by payment. This can result in a significant savings for your medical office with a large order.

We look forward to hearing from you soon. Please feel free to call your local representative, Mr. Nick Benedict, if you have any questions.

Sincerely,

Emma Bryant

Emma Bryant
Sales Manager

zz

Copy to Order Department

Figure 6-5 Modified Block Letter Style with Block Paragraphs

The Medical Example Company
4900 Drake Road • Bartlett, TN 38134-1492

June 18, 19--

CONFIDENTIAL

Take Charge Medical Industries
Attention Mrs. Martha Weller
255 Blue Hill Avenue
Boston, MA 02187-9561

Ladies and Gentlemen:

MODIFIED BLOCK MEDICAL LETTER STYLE

This letter is an example of the modified block medical letter style with block paragraphs. It is one of the most popular business letter styles in use today. You will note that the dateline and closing lines are indented and blocked at the center of the page. Mixed punctuation is frequently used with this letter style: a colon after the salutation and a comma after the complimentary close.

When the modified block medical letter style is used, letter production efficiency dictates that the dateline, the complimentary close, the company name, and the typed name and title of the originator be started at the center of the page.

This letter is also unusual in that it is loaded with special features. Normally, all illustrations here do not appear within one business letter. However, they are included here to show you their order within the medical business letter.

Sincerely,

THE MEDICAL EXAMPLE COMPANY

William McNae

William McNae
Chief Executive Officer

mos

Enclosures

cc Georgianna Stringer, DO

Please request additional information on business letter stationery from our home office.

Figure 6-6 Modified Block Letter Style with Indented Paragraphs

Bay Area Marine Supply
2232 Waterfront Drive
San Francisco, CA 31178-1564

April 10, 19—

Nancy A. List, D.O.
1754 Maple Ridge Road
Haslett, MI 48840-1616

Dear Dr. List

    It is a pleasure to confirm May 22 as the delivery date for your new 32-foot "Starlight" cruiser. The factory representatives assure me that the special options you ordered can be worked into their production schedule without any difficulty.

    Our original quotation of $198,600 is now a firm price. It is payable at the time title is transferred. Please let me know if you wish any assistance with financing.

    You have selected a fine boat; I hope you will spend many enjoyable hours aboard.

Very truly yours

Pasqual Otazu

Pasqual Otazu, President

mq

As you know, a member of our staff will be available to assist you on a shakedown cruise at your convenience anytime within 60 days of delivery.

Figure 6-7 Personal Business Letter

4408 Glen Rose Street
Fairfax, VA 22032-7429
January 15, 19—

Academic Advising Department
Santa Fe Community College
111 S.E. First Avenue
Gainesville, FL 33333-8495

Ladies and Gentlemen:

I am interested in enrolling in the Medical Technology training program offered at Santa Fe Community College.

I would appreciate receiving information regarding admission requirements and financial aid assistance available at Santa Fe. Also, please send me a copy of your college catalog containing information on course requirements for the Medical Technology program and course descriptions.

Do you have dormitories available on your campus? If not, are there student apartments near the campus? Since I will be coming from Virginia to attend Santa Fe, I will need some help in finding a place to live.

Thank you for your assistance.

Sincerely,

Karen McMeekin

Karen McMeekin

variable space in this method is the number of blank lines between the letterhead and dateline. The inside address is then typed on the fourth line below the date.

Table 6-2
Dateline Placement

	Five-Stroke Words in Letter Body	Date Placement
Small	Up to 125	Line 19
Medium	126-225	Line 16
Large	226-325	Line 13
Two-Page	326+	Line 13

Fixed Dateline. A second method of vertical placement of the date is called the fixed dateline. In this method the dateline is always typed on the second line below the last line of the printed letterhead. A fixed date placement is often used with word processing equipment.

6.15 Mailing Notations and Other Special Notations

Mailing notations (AIRMAIL, REGISTERED, CERTIFIED) and other special notations (PERSONAL, CONFIDENTIAL) are typed in all capital letters at the left margin a double space below the dateline.

6.16 Inside Address/Salutation

The *inside address* provides all the information needed for delivery of the medical business letter. The inside address includes name, title, company name, street number and name, city, two-letter state abbreviation, and ZIP Code. (For two-letter state abbreviations, see 6.29.) The inside address also provides the information needed to determine the correct salutation.

Following are several examples of inside addresses and appropriate salutations that may be used with each. Note that the city, state abbreviation, and ZIP Code are typed on one line. Two spaces (but no comma) separate the state abbreviation from the ZIP Code.

To an Individual (Colon after salutation indicates mixed punctuation):

Mr. Nelson Benedico
Tulane University
31 McAlister Drive
New Orleans, LA 85555-9776

Ms. Louise Adams
4 Linden Place
Cincinnati, OH 45227-2579

Dear Mr. Benedico:

Dear Ms. Adams:

To an Individual at a Business Address (Absence of punctuation after salutation indicates open punctuation):

Horace E. Traylor, M.D.
Instructional Resources
Los Angeles Pierce College
6201 Winnetka Avenue
Woodland, CA 91364-1903

Vice-President
School of Medicine
University of Miami
1600 N.W. 10 Avenue
Miami, FL 33136-2021

Dear Dr. Traylor

Dear Sir or Madam

To a Company or Organization:

The Upjohn Company
Pharmaceutical Sales Office
1974 Lashly Court
Snellville, GA 30278-1890

Ladies and Gentlemen:

Two-Line Address:

Miss Leota Schramm
Rogers City, MI 49779-7172

Dear Aunt Leota

Address with Apartment Number:

Mr. Nickson Benedico
7131 Wood Drive, Apt. 151
Austin, TX 78731-6634

Dear Nicky

Two People, Different Addresses:

Ralph Tejeda, M.D.   and   Ileana Gonzalez, D.O.
P.O. Box 2143   4408 Glen Rose Street
Riverview Road   Fairfax, VA 22032-2763
Riverton, WY 82501-5998

Dear Drs. Tejeda and Gonzalez:

Two People, Same Address:

- Eliminate official titles, unless they are short and can fit on the same line with the name.

- Eliminate the department name, unless both are from the same department.

- On individual envelopes, type full addresses.

        Ms. Pam Stringer
        Mr. Tom Petersen
        Legal Services Association
        1150 N. Franklin
        Dearborn, MI 48128-2881

        Dear Pam and Tom:

Titles:

- Change the position of titles to balance the inside address.

        Dr. Elaine Dillard, Director
        Cornwall Medical Center
        15432 Kit Lane
        Fort Worth, TX 75240-5999

        Dr. Garth Reeves
        Vice-President
        Cornwall Medical Center
        15432 Kit Lane
        Fort Worth, TX 75240-9954

        Robert McCabe, M.D.
        Vice-President and
          General Manager
        Cornwall Medical Center
        15432 Kit Lane
        Fort Worth, TX 75240-6677

Single Digit Addresses:

- When house or building numbers consist of a *1*, spell out *one*. Use numbers for all other single digit addresses.

        One Woodward Avenue
        3 Maple Lane

Room, Suite, Building in Address:

- Long company names can be divided and put on two lines.

Mr. Alan Courtney
Attorney at Law
429 Broad Street, Suite 13
Richmond, VA 23219-1543

Columbus Employees
   Federal Credit Union
Penobscot Building, Room 118
1800 King Avenue
Columbus, OH 48216-1603

Dear Mr. Courtney:

                            Ladies and Gentlemen:

Husband and Wife:

        Dr. and Mrs. Jules Avery
        Plaza Medical Center
        2050 Massachusetts Avenue
        Washington, DC 20503-8181

        Dear Dr. and Mrs. Avery:

Foreign Country:

- Type the name of a foreign country in all caps.

        Mr. William McNae
        Hert Medical Interiors, Ltd.
        27 Monks Close
        Leeds, York ALY-372
        UNITED KINGDOM

        Dear Mr. McNae:

In Care Of:

Alberta Goodman, D.O.
In care of John Roueche, D.O.
University of Texas at Austin
Austin, TX 78731-1023

                      or   c/o John Roueche, D.O.

Dear Dr. Goodman:

6.17   Attention Line

An *attention line* is often used to route a letter to a particular person when a letter is addressed to a company. The attention line indicates that the letter concerns company business and that the writer prefers that the letter be handled by the individual named in the attention line (or by another individual in the same position if the person named is no longer with the company). The attention line is typed as the second line of the inside address. Note that the salutation agrees with the inside address, not the attention line.

```
Carolina Labs                      Alberto Medical Supplies
Attention Sally Buxton, M.D.       ATTENTION Dan Derrico, D.O.
1005 Ala Lililoi Street            2525 W. Armitage Avenue
Honolulu, HI  96818-0017           Melrose Park, IL  60164-5361

Ladies and Gentlemen:              Ladies and Gentlemen:
```

6.18   Subject Line

When a *subject line* is included, it serves as a title to the body of the letter. It should be typed a double space below the salutation at the left margin. With the Modified Block letter, the subject line may be centered, begin at the left margin, or be indented five spaces to align with the first line of indented paragraphs. The words *SUBJECT* or *RE* are sometimes used with the subject line, but are not required. The subject line can be typed in all caps, in capitals and lowercase, or in capitals and lowercase underlined. A double space follows the subject line, before beginning the body of the letter.

```
Detroit, MI  48219-1770

Dear Dr. Stringer:

     ANNUAL PEDIATRICIANS CONFERENCE
```

```
Detroit, MI  48219-7052

Dear Dr. Stringer:

SUBJECT: Annual Pediatricians Conference
```

```
Detroit, MI 48219-7052

Dear Dr. Stringer:

    RE: Annual Pediatricians Conference
```

6.19 Body

The message of your medical letter is carried to the reader by the *body* of the letter. Each paragraph should be single-spaced with a double space between paragraphs. Paragraphs begin at the left margin (except in the Modified Block with Indented Paragraphs style, where paragraphs are indented five spaces).

Try to balance paragraph size, and write at least two paragraphs in a letter. A very short letter (six lines or less) may be double-spaced, or extra blank lines may be inserted between letter parts to achieve balance.

Quoted or tabulated material within a letter is set off by a double space before and after the quotation, and by a five-space indent from each margin.

6.20 Complimentary Close, Company Name, and Signature Lines

A recent survey of businesses found that the majority used "Very truly yours" or "Sincerely" for the *complimentary close*. Two other popular complimentary closes were "Sincerely yours" and "Yours very truly." Type the complimentary close at the left margin in Block style letters, and begin at the center in Modified Block style. The complimentary close should be typed a double space below the body of the letter. Capitalize only the first letter of the first word in the complimentary close. With mixed punctuation, type a comma after the complimentary close, but with open punctuation, use no punctuation.

If letterhead is not used, the company name is typed in all capital letters a double space after the complimentary close. The company name begins in the same place (left margin or center) as the complimentary close.

The *signature lines* show the writer's name, and often include the writer's title or department or both. They fall four lines below the complimentary close (or company name if it is included). The signature line begins in the same place (left margin or center) as the complimentary close.

Sincerely,	Very truly yours
PERSUTTI ASSOCIATES	PRIDE INTERNATIONAL
Delphine Persutti President	Diana Campoamor, Ph.D. Dean of Students

- Titles may be on the same line as the writer's name, or on the following line.

- Titles of Miss, Ms., or Mrs. may be shown in the typed or written signature. Parentheses are optional.

Sincerely yours,	Sincerely,
Miss Tomoko Sumida Manager	Dr. Ronald Garson Vice-President

Hyphenated Last Names. Some hyphenated names have special significance in Hispanic cultures. Hyphenated names such as Hernandez-Fumero are used by Hispanic males and females. The two names represent the two sides of the person's family, the father's and the mother's. Both names are used to indicate a pride in heritage. When a hyphenated Hispanic name is used, the signature will always reflect the same hyphenation.

>Sincerely yours,
>
>
>Aida Hernandez-Fumero
>Public Relations Director

Hyphenated last names are also used by many married females of other cultures to include both the maiden and married names. Thus, if Miss Bonnie Landsea married Mr. Geoff Gathercole, she would become:

>Bonnie Landsea-Gathercole
>Mrs. Bonnie Landsea-Gathercole
>Mrs. Geoff Landsea-Gathercole

This usage also reflects a pride in family heritage. The signature may or may not reflect the hyphenated name.

6.21   Reference Initials

Reference initials identify the typist and sometimes the writer of medical correspondence. They are typed a double space below the final signature line at the left margin. Reference initials are typed in a variety of ways:

- Indicating the typist:

    ```
    kds    zz    MAP
    ```

- Indicating the writer (first initials) and the typist:

    ```
    ALR:kss    TRD/POE    SR:cm
    ```

    The writer's initials are included in this way only if the writer's name is not typed.

- Sometimes the writer of the letter (if different than the signer) is indicated this way:

    ```
    CRWhite/pg
    ```

6.22   Enclosure Notation

When any additional information is to be enclosed in the envelope with the medical correspondence, an enclosure notation should be used. This notation is typed at the left margin a double space after the reference initials. Enclosure notations are typed in a variety of ways:

Enclosure	Enclosures (2)
Enc.	Enc. 2

Check Enclosed

6.23   Copy Notation

When copies of a letter are to be sent to individuals other than the addressee, a copy notation should be typed at the left margin, a double space below the enclosure notation. (Note: *c* means *copy*, *pc* means *photocopy*, and *cc* means *carbon copy*)

c Dr. Hansen
  Dr. Kelly
	pc Research Department
	   Personnel

Also used:

PC: Mr. Maxwell Kamin Dr. Joan Schaeffer	Copy to Purchasing

Sometimes the letter writer wants to send a copy of a medical letter to someone without the addressee's knowledge. In this case, a *blind copy* notation should be used. Type the following indication on the file copy:

>   bc: Mr. Reuben Goldstein
>   Legal Department

It is helpful to indicate when enclosures are (or are not) sent to those receiving copies:

>   pc (w/enclosures) Dr. Harriet Spivak
>   Dr. Charlotte Gallogly
>
>   cc Dr. Harriet Spivak (w/enclosures)
>   Dr. Charlotte Gallogly (w/o enclosures)

6.24 File Copies

Copies of all medical correspondence should be available in the medical office. Copies can be stored on paper, or electronically on a magnetic disk or in a shared logic system.

Paper file copies are still the most common means of storage in medical offices. Copies are made with carbon paper, NCR (no carbon required) paper, or on the office photocopier. Some medical offices have special sheets with simplified letterheads for copies sent outside the medical office. Paper copies are filed for quick retrieval in a metal cabinet.

Electronic file copies are made automatically when medical letters keyboarded on a word processor or computer are saved. While the original medical letter is typed using the printer (and copies are usually made on a photocopier), the office file copy is stored electronically. This saves office storage space and allows for future electronic transmission of the document to other medical offices. The impact of the electronic office is discussed in detail in Chapters 13 and 14.

6.25 Additional Pages

When a letter extends to a second page, use a plain piece of bond paper of the same quality as the original letterhead. Using the same side margins, the second page should begin on line seven with a heading which indicates to whom the letter was written.

>   Schaeffer Medical Research Group
>   Page 2
>   September 15, 19—

or

Schaeffer Medical Research Group 2 September 15, 19—

Following the second page heading, triple-space and resume typing the body of the letter.

- Do not divide a paragraph between pages unless two lines remain on the first page and at least two lines of the same paragraph begin the second page.

- Leave a uniform bottom margin of at least one inch at the bottom of all letter pages.

- Do not hyphenate the final word on a page.

- Do not use the second page to type only the complimentary close and following lines. At least two lines of the final paragraph should begin the second page.

6.26 Typing an Interoffice Memorandum

Letters sent to individuals within the same medical organization are often typed as interoffice memorandums. This allows for the use of less expensive stationery, and immediately shows that the correspondence is from within the organization.

Interoffice memorandums are typed on memorandum forms or on plain paper. The headings TO, FROM, DATE, and SUBJECT always begin the memorandum. The subject line may or may not be typed in all capital letters. There are no complimentary close or signature lines in an interoffice memorandum. The writer signs (using name or initials) next to the writer's name at the top. Reference initials, enclosure notations, and copy notations remain the same as in medical business letters. (See Figure 6-8)

6.27 Composing for the Doctor's Signature

The medical office worker should become familiar with typical answers to routine medical correspondence. In the electronic office, sample paragraphs can be stored for later rearrangement and use in medical correspondence. It will be helpful to the doctor if you can draft routine medical correspondence. The doctor will then review, make any necessary corrections, and sign the final document.

Figure 6-8 Medical Interoffice Memorandum

April 10, 19--

TO: Jeff Brezner
          Facilities Department

FROM: Marie Hydress MH   [NOTE: Courtesy titles (Dr.,
          Personnel Department   Mr., Ms., Mrs., and Miss)
                                          are not used by the
DATE: April 10, 19--   writer.]

SUBJECT: EMPLOYEE PICNIC

Thank you for agreeing to serve on our committee to organize the employee picnic next month. Because of the group of individuals who will be working on the arrangements, I am sure our picnic this year will be the best ever!

Enclosed are the following items from last year's efforts:

          Planning Committee Report
          Picnic Budget
          Picnic Employee Flyer
          Picnic Program
          Picnic Evaluation

The first meeting of our planning committee will be in the executive dining room on Tuesday, July 17, 19--, at 2:00 p.m. My secretary will be calling you to confirm your attendance at this meeting.

Bring your best ideas -- let's make this picnic one that will be long remembered.

mos

Enclosures

c Dr. Kevin Donovan

OUTGOING MAIL

6.28 Preparation of Envelopes

Prepare envelopes for outgoing mail before presenting the letter to the writer for signature. Each envelope should include the return address of the writer, the complete address of the person or organization that is to receive the letter, and any special mailing notations. Both of these addresses on the envelope should contain the two-letter state abbreviation and ZIP Code. The United States Postal Service prefers that envelope addresses be typed in all capital letters with no punctuation between the two-letter state abbreviation and the ZIP Code.

6.29 Two-Letter State and Provincial Abbreviations

The following table shows the names of the states, districts, and territories of the United States and the two-letter abbreviations of each that are used with ZIP Codes.

Table 6-3
Two-Letter State, District, and Territory Abbreviations

Name	Abbreviation
Alabama	AL
Alaska	AK
Arizona	AZ
Arkansas	AR
California	CA
Colorado	CO
Connecticut	CT
Delaware	DE
District of Columbia	DC
Florida	FL
Georgia	GA
Guam	GU
Hawaii	HI
Idaho	ID
Illinois	IL
Indiana	IN
Iowa	IA
Kansas	KS

Table 6-3 (continued)

Kentucky	KY
Louisiana	LA
Maine	ME
Maryland	MD
Massachusetts	MA
Michigan	MI
Minnesota	MN
Mississippi	MS
Missouri	MO
Montana	MT
Nebraska	NE
Nevada	NV
New Hampshire	NH
New Jersey	NJ
New Mexico	NM
New York	NY
North Carolina	NC
North Dakota	ND
Ohio	OH
Oklahoma	OK
Oregon	OR
Pennsylvania	PA
Puerto Rico	PR
Rhode Island	RI
South Carolina	SC
South Dakota	SD
Tennessee	TN
Texas	TX
Utah	UT
Vermont	VT
Virgin Islands	VI
Virginia	VA
Washington	WA
West Virginia	WV
Wisconsin	WI
Wyoming	WY

Medical Communications

The following table shows the names of the Canadian provinces and the two-letter abbreviations of each that are used with ZIP Codes.

Table 6-4
Two-Letter Provincial Abbreviations

Names	Abbreviations
Alberta	AB
British Columbia	BC
Manitoba	MB
New Brunswick	NB
Newfoundland	NF
Northwest Territories	NT
Nova Scotia	NS
Ontario	ON
Prince Edward Island	PE
Quebec	PQ
Saskatchewan	SK
Yukon Territory	YT

6.30   Return Address

Letterhead envelopes have the name and address of your medical office printed in the upper left corner of the envelope. It may, however, be necessary for you to type the name of the letter writer, department, or the account number (if you work for a large medical office). This information should be typed above the printed return address.

For personal business correspondence, or if your medical office does not use printed envelopes, the return address should be typed a double space from the top edge of the envelope and three to four spaces from the left edge.

6.31   Mailing Address

The mailing address on a large envelope should be typed five spaces to the left of the horizontal center, and on line 14. On a small envelope, type the address ten spaces left of center, and on line 12.

6.32   Nine-Digit Expanded ZIP Code

The U.S. Postal Service has added four more digits to the standard five-digit ZIP Code. Most medical offices have now been informed of their new expanded ZIP Code. This expanded ZIP Code will allow faster processing of all mail, which should result in faster delivery. This is important in view of the larger volume of mail processed each year by the Postal Service. If you have any questions about your office's ZIP Code, contact your local post office.

6.33 Envelope Notations

Notations that are intended for the receivers of mail are called addressee notations. These notations are used by the person(s) delivering mail within the medical office and include messages such as PERSONAL, CONFIDENTIAL, HOLD FOR ARRIVAL, and PLEASE FORWARD. Addressee notations should be typed in all capital letters a triple space below the return address and three to four spaces from the left edge.

Mailing notations, those mailing directions intended for the U.S. Postal Service, include REGISTERED, RETURN RECEIPT REQUESTED, and SPECIAL DELIVERY. Such notations identify special mailing requirements for postal personnel and should be typed a triple space below the postage stamp (or postage meter mark) in all capital letters.

Figure 6-9, page 102, shows the correct way to type both small and large business envelopes with a variety of mailing notations.

6.34 Folding Business Letters

The correct procedure for folding business letters and inserting them into envelopes varies according to the size of the envelope you are using. Figure 6-10, page 103, shows how to fold a business letter for large and small business envelopes. Also shown are illustrations for folding business correspondence for use with window envelopes. Make certain the complete address shows clearly through the window of the envelope after insertion.

6.35 Metered Mail

In a large medical office, postage will probably be added to envelopes by a postage metering machine. This machine adds different amounts of postage depending on the weight of the envelope or package being mailed. To make rapid metering easier, leave envelope flaps open and make sure all addresses face the same way. The metering machine automatically seals all envelopes as it adds postage. Confidential mail can be sealed before sending it to the mailroom, if desired. To avoid machine damage, letter envelopes containing bulky items, such as paper clips, should be sealed and marked *Hand Stamp* by the originating office.

102 Medical Communications

Figure 6-9 Envelope Address Placement

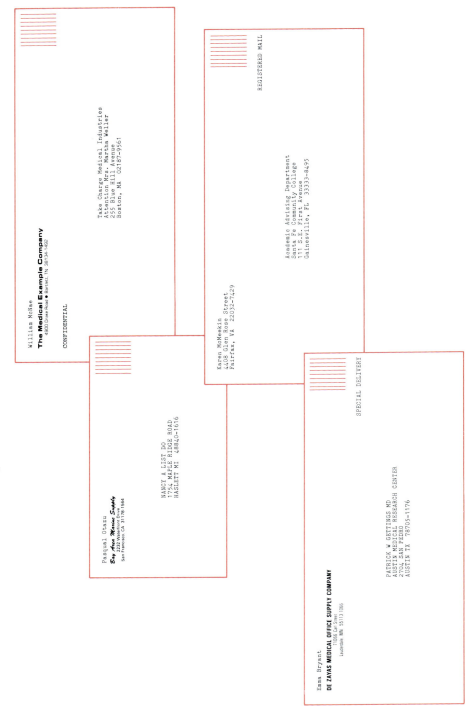

Chapter 6—Medical Correspondence 103

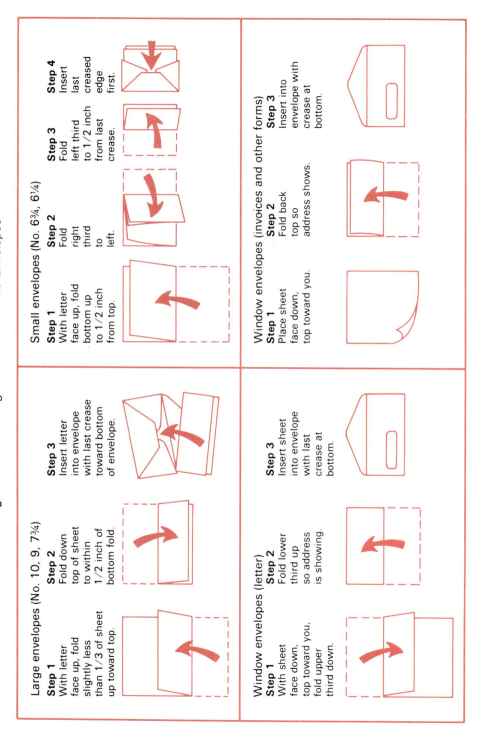

Figure 6-10 Folding Letters for Various Envelopes

6.36 Classes of Mail

First-class mail is delivered by the fastest transportation available. It is the most expensive class of mail delivery. For mail delivered within the United States, it is no longer necessary to specify "Air Mail," since all first-class mail is now sent by air. First-class mail generally includes letters, post cards, business reply mail, greeting cards, bills, checks, money orders, reports, and manuscripts.

Second-class mail is generally used for newspapers and magazines, while advertising material is usually sent by third-class mail. Fourth-class mail is generally used for mailing packages weighing 16 ounces or more.

Each of these classes of mail has special requirements regarding size and weight. For specific information, consult your local post office.

6.37 Special Mailing Services

Special mailing services and delivery schedules are available through the Postal Service and through private letter and parcel carriers. Consult your local telephone book for a complete list of mail delivery services. Some of the currently available mailing services include overnight delivery and special delivery; insurance for letters and packages; certificates of mailing, which prove you mailed something; and certified mail with a return receipt, which proves mail was delivered and provides you with the signature of the individual receiving the mail. Other available services include registered mail (for items that cannot be replaced or are valued at more than $400), COD (cash on delivery), money orders, and mail forwarding. Each of these services has restrictions and requirements on time, size, and weight. Check with your local post office or private mail carrier for details.

7

Medical Office Files

TYPES OF MEDICAL OFFICE FILES

Medical records, ledger cards, general correspondence, research reports, tax records, and magazine articles related to the physician's specialty are typical documents which must be filed in a medical office. The alphabetic and numeric filing methods are commonly used for filing patient records, while the alphabetic, numeric, geographic, and subject methods are used for other materials.

7.1 Patient Files

Medical Records. When the alphabetic method is used for medical records, materials are filed according to letters of the alphabet. When the numeric method is used, materials are filed according to a preassigned patient number. While the alphabetic method involves fewer steps than the numeric method, the numeric method provides greater confidentiality. Materials within a record may be filed in chronological order (by date), or they may be filed according to type: for example, all blood test results might be filed together, all EKG results together, and all urinalysis reports together (see Sections 5.17 and 5.18, page 73.).

Ledger Cards. Ledger cards are filed in alphabetic order and stored in a separate file. They are retrieved as necessary for posting of patient charges, credits, and adjustments (see Section 11.2, page 168.).

7.2 Inactive and Closed Patient Files

When a patient has not visited the physician for an extended period, the medical record is moved to the *inactive files*. Most physicians consider a patient to be inactive after two to three years. *Closed files* contain the medical records of patients who are no longer under the care of the physician because they have moved, changed doctors, or died.

Inactive and closed files are kept indefinitely because they provide protection against medical malpractice claims. Malpractice suits can be filed several years following the disputed treatment. The laws of each state regarding the statute of limitations (how long after a disputed action a claim can be made) can be a guide in determining how long the inactive records should be kept.

7.3 Miscellaneous Correspondence Files

Letters, memos, reports, and other general documents not directly related to patients are filed according to subject in a separate *miscellaneous correspondence file* (see Section 7.28, p. 124). Examples of miscellaneous correspondence include letters regarding the lease of office space, price lists for medical supply houses, professional meeting announcements, and tax records.

A folder labeled "Miscellaneous Correspondence" is used for any subject for which there is no individual folder. The correspondence is clipped together by subject and arranged in alphabetic order within the folder. When there are more than five items about a single subject, (1) an individual folder is prepared, (2) the materials are transferred to the new folder, and (3) the folder is then merged with the other individual folders.

The individual folders are filed in alphabetic order with the miscellaneous folder stored at the back of the file.

7.4 Research Files

Medical research is filed according to the subject or geographic methods. Research about allergies, for example, might be filed according to the name of the allergy, such as "hay fever" or "poison ivy," or according to the geographic areas of the country where the allergy is found. Sometimes both the subject and geographic methods are used in a research file. Figure 7-1 illustrates a research file with allergy names as subjects and regions of the country as subcategories. The subject and geographic categories are arranged in alphabetic order. The numeric method also can be used to identify folders in a research file (see Section 7.29.).

7.5 Automated Files

Computer technology lends itself to the storage of medical files, including medical records, accounting, and research records (see Chapter 14). As with physical storage of materials, the methods of computer filing are alphabetic, numeric, subject, and geographic. Several software companies offer systems for medical record keeping which are compatible with popular computers.

Chapter 7—Medical Office Files 107

Figure 7-1 Research File Using the Subject, Geographic, and Alphabetic Filing Methods.

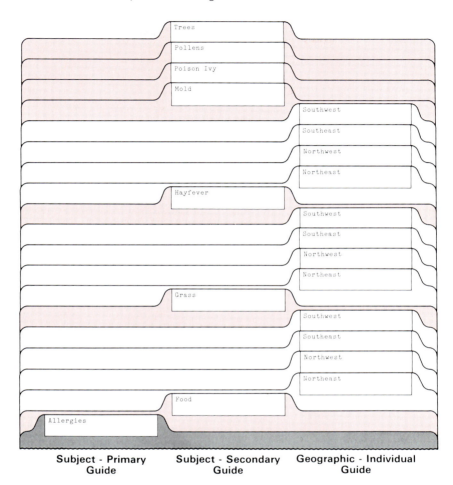

7.6 Microfiche and Microfilm

Large medical facilities often use *microfiche* or *microfilm* to store inactive and closed records. Since a sheet of microfiche is about the size of a three-by-five-inch index card and holds 96 pages of information, records for several patients can be filmed on one microfiche sheet and stored in much less space than would be necessary for conventional records. Microfiche cameras reduce and film a record; a microfiche reader enlarges the record for viewing. Microfiche are filed inside paper jackets and stored in trays. A microfiche is shown in Figure 7-2. Microfilm is a roll of film on which records are reduced and stored. It is similar to microfiche, except that the film is on a roll instead of a sheet. Microfilm is viewed through a microfilm reader. A roll of microfilm is shown in Figure 7-3.

Figure 7-2 Microfiche

Figure 7-3 Microfilm

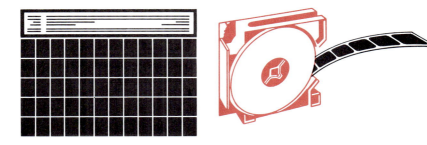

Because of advances in computer technology, records can be stored directly onto microfilm or microfiche from a computer or a word processor. Records can also be sent to an outside filming company for photographing on microfilm or microfiche; however, some physicians prefer not to use the services of an outside company because of the confidential nature of medical records.

ALPHABETIC INDEXING

The alphabet is basic to all four methods of filing: alphabetic, numeric, subject, and geographic. Several standard rules apply for filing by the alphabetic method.

7.7   Rule 1: Order of Indexing Units

For filing purposes, the parts of an individual's name are called indexing units. The surname, or last name, is identified as the first indexing unit; the first name or initial is identified as the second unit; and the middle name or initial is identified as the third unit.

Names	Unit 1	Unit 2	Unit 3
Samuel Arthur Clark	Clark	Samuel	Arthur
Terry Alaine Clark	Clark	Terry	Alaine
Terry Elaine Clark	Clark	Terry	Elaine
Marcy Roderick	Roderick	Marcy	
Samuel Earl Watkins	Watkins	Samuel	Earl

7.8 Rule 2: Names of Businesses

Names of businesses, institutions, and organizations are indexed in the order in which the name is written. If a business name includes more than one unit of an individual's name, the individual's name is indexed as written. Abbreviations such as *Co., Inc.,* and *Ltd.,* are also indexed as written.

Names	Unit 1	Unit 2	Unit 3	Unit 4
Clinical Supply Company	Clinical	Supply	Company	
John Martin Pediatrics	John	Martin	Pediatrics	
Martin Prosthetics Company	Martin	Prosthetics	Company	
Otto Quantock Flower Shop	Otto	Quantock	Flower	Shop
Quantock Orthopedic Supplies	Quantock	Orthopedic	Supplies	
Valery Wiley Flower Shop	Valery	Wiley	Flower	Shop

7.9 Rule 3: Symbols and Small Words

Symbols and small words are also used as indexing units. These words and symbols include *a, an, and, the, in, of, #,* and *&*. Symbols are considered as spelled in full. When *the* is the first word of a business name, it is considered to be the last indexing unit.

Names	Unit 1	Unit 2	Unit 3	Unit 4
Harris of Atlanta	Harris	of	Atlanta	
Palmer & Palmer Labs	Palmer	and	Palmer	Labs
The Sands Ambulance Service	Sands	Ambulance	Service	The
Thomas and Sons Oxygen	Thomas	and	Sons	Oxygen
Walters & Walters Realty	Walters	and	Walters	Realty

7.10 Rule 4: Initials and Abbreviations

Initials and abbreviations of business and personal names are indexed as written. The use of hyphens, periods, or parentheses are unimportant and do not influence the indexing order.

Names	Unit 1	Unit 2	Unit 3	Unit 4	Unit 5
A.B.C Radiology Co.	ABC	Radiology	Co		
C & D Drug Co.	C	and	D	Drug	Co
F. Garamond, Inc.	F	Garamond	Inc		
The Wm. A. Williams Corp.	Wm	A	Williams	Corp	The
Wm. A. Wms. Assoc.	Wm	A	Wms	Assoc	

7.11 Rule 5: Possessives

The apostrophe is no longer considered when indexing possessives. The apostrophe is disregarded and possessives are indexed as written. *Harper's* is indexed as *Harpers* and *Manns'* is indexed as *Manns*.

Names	Unit 1	Unit 2	Unit 3	Unit 4
Kimber's Ophthalmologists	Kimbers	Ophthalmologists		
Markhams' Limited	Markhams	Limited		
Markham's Uniforms	Markhams	Uniforms		
Romer's Insurance Co.	Romers	Insurance	Co	
Ruble & Ruble Agency	Ruble	and	Ruble	Agency
Ruble's Nursing Home	Rubles	Nursing	Home	

7.12 Rule 6: Titles

A title is considered as the last indexing unit. If it appears with only one personal name, the name and title are indexed as written. Business names are indexed as written.

Names	Unit 1	Unit 2	Unit 3
Dr. Ester Diaz	Diaz	Ester	Dr
Doctor Watson	Doctor	Watson	
Father Watson	Father	Watson	
Rev. Joseph Mendel	Mendel	Joseph	Rev
Mr. Carl Coiffures	Mr	Carl	Coiffures
Prince George Opticals	Prince	George	Opticals
Professor Mendel	Professor	Mendel	
Carla Walgreen, M.D.	Walgreen	Carla	MD
Mr. Franklin Watson	Watson	Franklin	Mr

7.13 Rule 7: Married Women

A married woman's name is indexed as used. Some married women use their husband's last name and their own first name and middle name or initial. Other married women use their husband's last name as well as his first name and middle name or initial. In either case, the last name is the first indexing unit, the first name is the second indexing unit, and the middle name or initial is the third indexing unit.

Some married women use a combination of their own last name and their husband's last name, plus their first name and middle name or initial. The compound last name is considered as one indexing unit. The first name is the second unit, and the middle name or initial is the third unit (see Section 7.19). When a married woman is known by more than one name, all forms of the name are cross-referenced (see Section 7.23).

Names	Unit 1	Unit 2	Unit 3	Unit 4
Mrs. Nobel D. Brown (Mrs. Fay Brown)	Brown	Nobel	D	Mrs
Ms. Alice Marie Lunkin	Lunkin	Alice	Marie	Ms
Mrs. Carl Henry Sanders (Mrs. Ellen Theresa Sanders)	Sanders	Carl	Henry	Mrs

Names	Unit 1	Unit 2	Unit 3	Unit 4
Dr. Carmen C. Sanders	Sanders	Carmen	C	Dr
Mrs. Sarah Edna Sanders	Sanders	Sarah	Edna	Mrs
Ms. Althea Sanders-Smith	SandersSmith	Althea	Ms	

7.14 Rule 8: Foreign Language Prefixes

A foreign language prefix is considered to be a part of the business name or personal name which follows it. Capitalization or spacing between the prefix and the root word does not influence the indexing order. Examples of foreign language prefixes include *De, Di, Du, L', Las, O', Van,* and *Van Der.*

Names	Unit 1	Unit 2	Unit 3	Unit 4
Miss Donna Di George	DiGeorge	Donna	Miss	
Dr. Sarah Jane Du Pont	DuPont	Sarah	Jane	Dr
Sarah M. Dupont, M.D.	Dupont	Sarah	M	MD
Sarah R. DuPont, Ph.D.	DuPont	Sarah	R	PhD
MacDonald Druggists	MacDonald	Druggists		
McDonald Drugs	McDonald	Drugs		
Rev. DuPont	Rev	DuPont		
S. McDonald & Sons	S	McDonald	and	Sons
Lucille Vanhook	Vanhook	Lucille		
William Van Hook Optical Co.	William	VanHook	Optical	Co

7.15 Rule 9: Identical Names

When several names of individuals or businesses are the same, addresses are considered for filing. Addresses are indexed first by city, then by state (if city name is duplicated), then by street name and address or building number. Addresses and building numbers are indexed in ascending order.

Chapter 7—Medical Office Files

The seniority designations *Junior* (*Jr.*) and *Senior* (*Sr.*) are considered in alphabetic order. The seniority designations *II*, *III*, and *IV* are considered in numeric order.

Names	Unit 1	Unit 2	Unit 3	Unit 4	Unit 5	Unit 6	Unit 7
Metro Ambulance Service Atlanta, Georgia	Metro	Ambulance	Service	Atlanta	Georgia		
Metro Ambulance Service Columbus, Georgia	Metro	Ambulance	Service	Columbus	Georgia		
Metro Ambulance Service Columbus, Ohio	Metro	Ambulance	Service	Columbus	Ohio		

Metro Ambulance Service
   312 Archer Place
   Dallas, Texas
	Metro	Ambulance	Service	Dallas	Texas	Archer Place	312

Metro Ambulance Service
   1802 Peyton Lane
   Dallas, Texas
	Metro	Ambulance	Service	Dallas	Texas	Peyton Lane	1802

Metro Ambulance Service
   2405 Peyton Lane
   Dallas, Texas
	Metro	Ambulance	Service	Dallas	Texas	Peyton Lane	2405

Metro Ambulance Service Manchester, Iowa	Metro	Ambulance	Service	Manchester	Iowa		
Arthur Sylvester	Sylvester	Arthur					
Arthur Sylvester Jr.	Sylvester	Arthur	Jr.				
Arthur Sylvester Sr.	Sylvester	Arthur	Sr.				
Francisco Toros	Toros	Francisco					
Francisco Toros II	Toros	Francisco	II				
Francisco Toros III	Toros	Francisco	III				

7.16 Rule 10: Numerals in Business Names

A numeral which is part of a business name is written as a single word and indexed as a single unit. Arabic numerals and Roman numerals are filed sequentially before alphabetic characters.

Names	Unit 1	Unit 2	Unit 3	Unit 4
9th Avenue Garage	9	Avenue	Garage	
900 Sounds, Inc.	900	Sounds	Inc	
1980s Ambulance Service	1980s	Ambulance	Service	
20-20 Vision Associates	2020	Vision	Associates	
9000 Physicians Group	9000	Physicians	Group	
VII Systems, Inc.	VII	Systems	Inc	
IX Hills Country Club	IX	Hills	Country	Club
Nine Hundred Block Drugs	Nine	Hundred	Block	Drugs
Nine Street Orthopedic Supplies	Nine	Street	Orthopedic	Supplies
Nineteen Hundred Club	Nineteen	Hundred	Club	
Ninth Street Emergency Center	Ninth	Street	Emergency	Center

7.17 Rule 11: Organizations and Institutions

Names of organizations and institutions are indexed as written.

Names	Unit 1	Unit 2	Unit 3	Unit 4
American Cancer Society	American	Cancer	Society	
American Medical Association	American	Medical	Association	
Commission for the Arts	Commission	for	the	Arts
First Baptist Church	First	Baptist	Church	
Franklin State Bank	Franklin	State	Bank	
Motel Six	Motel	Six		
National Association of Radiologists	National	Association	of	Radiologists

7.18 Rule 12: Separated Single Words

Separate parts of words considered by the dictionary to be a single word are indexed as written in the business name. If the word is separated in the business name it should be indexed as separate units. Hyphens, capitalizations, and spacing are disregarded.

Names	Unit 1	Unit 2	Unit 3	Unit 4
Inter State Listing Service	Inter	State	Listing	Service
Interstate Blood Bank	Interstate	Blood	Bank	
North East Optical Supplies	North	East	Optical	Supplies
Northeast Ambulance Service	Northeast	Ambulance	Service	
South-side Pharmacy	Southside	Pharmacy		
Dr. Raymond Southside	Southside	Raymond	Dr	
Southwest Ohio Medical Group	Southwest	Ohio	Medical	Group
South-West Ortho Center	SouthWest	Ortho	Center	

7.19 Rule 13: Compound Names

Parts of compound business names separated by a space are indexed as individual units. Hyphens are disregarded and the parts are considered a single unit. Forms of the word *Saint*, such as *San* and *Sainte*, are considered prefixes and are indexed as part of the names that follow. (See Rule 8: Section 7.14)

Names	Unit 1	Unit 2	Unit 3	Unit 4	Unit 5
A-B-C Radiology	ABC	Radiology			
C & D Drug Company	C	and	D	Drug	Company
Geo. Reynolds Corrective Footwear	Geo	Reynolds	Corrective	Footwear	
Mason-Reynolds Accounting Service	MasonReynolds	Accounting	Service		
Pan American Airlines	Pan	American	Airlines		
Arnold Saint James	SaintJames	Arnold			

Names	Unit 1	Unit 2	Unit 3	Unit 4	Unit 5
San Francisco Medical Center	SanFrancisco	Medical	Center		
Santa Fe Railroad	SantaFe	Railroad			
Wm. A. Wms. & Sons	Wm	A	Wms	and	Sons

7.20   Rule 14: Coined Words, Unusual Words

Coined or unusual words are indexed as written. Hyphens are disregarded.

Names	Unit 1	Unit 2	Unit 3	Unit 4
A-1 Orthopedic Supplies	A1	Orthopedic	Supplies	
The Apotha Carry	Apotha	Carry	The	
Cash 'N Carry Supply	Cash	N	Carry	Supply
Lu-yin Cheng	Cheng	Luyin		
Da-O-Da Amusement Park	DaODa	Amusement	Park	
Opti Care Center	Opti	Care	Center	
Pepto-Bismol®	PeptoBismol			
Shur-Fit Optical	ShurFit	Optical		

7.21   Rule 15: Government Names

All government agencies, both domestic (in the United States) and foreign (from another country), are indexed according to political divisions. The name of the government body is indexed first (country, state, city) and is followed by the other units in descending order of importance (department, bureau, division, agency). The words *Bureau of, Department of, County of,* etc., are eliminated unless needed for clarity. Sometimes the words *United States Government* are understood to be part of a name but are not written in the name. They should always be considered as Units 1, 2, and 3 for filing purposes.

Rule 15: Government Names

Names	Unit 1	Unit 2	Unit 3	Unit 4	Unit 5	Unit 6	Unit 7	Unit 8	Unit 9
State of Georgia Department of Human Resources	Georgia	State	of	Human	Resources	Department	of		
Hamilton County Department of Public Works Cincinnati, Ohio	Hamilton	County	Public	Works	Department	of	Cincinnati	Ohio	
Republic of South Korea Ministry of Education	South	Korea	Republic	of	Education	Ministry	of		
Board of Education Sycamore School District Cincinnati, Ohio	Sycamore	School	District	Education	Board	of	Cincinnati	Ohio	
United States Government Department of Commerce	United	States	Government	Commerce	Department	of			
U.S. Dept. of Health and Human Services	United	States	Government	Health	and	Human	Services	Department	of

7.22 Alphabetic Filing Guides and Tabs

Primary file guides, made of heavy cardboard or plastic, identify the broad categories of a file. In an alphabetic file, primary guides usually divide the alphabet into 26 sections, one primary guide for each letter of the alphabet. The primary guides are placed in the first position of the file shelf (at the top) or file drawer (at the far left). Secondary guides subdivide the alphabet into smaller parts; for example, the primary guide *A* may be subdivided into *Aa-Al* and *Am-Az*. Secondary guides are placed in second position of the file shelf or file drawer. File folders with their individual captions often are placed in third position. For the medical office which wishes to further subdivide folders, guides are available for fourth and fifth positions. Color coding aids in locating folders, reducing the need for some of the secondary guides used in the past (see Section 7.37, page 128). Figure 7-4 illustrates an alphabetic file with guides and tabs.

Figure 7-4 Alphabetic File with Guides and Tabs

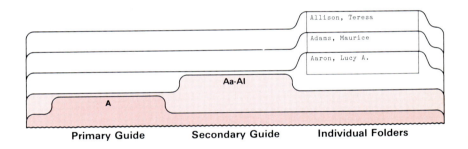

7.23 Cross-Referencing

A cross-reference card is used when a name might be indexed in more than one way. Foreign names, names of married women, unusual business names, hyphenated names, multiple business names, abbreviated or single-letter names, and names which may be spelled several ways are examples of situations in which a cross-reference card should be made.

If more than one name is associated with an individual, firm, or agency, the original card lists the name which is the most likely means of identification. A second, and perhaps third, card is used to show other names by which the individual, firm, or agency might be identified.

Figure 7-5 Cross-Reference for a Foreign Name

```
Cheng, Ai-ling

Ai-ling Cheng
505 South Perkins Drive
Memphis, TN  38117-3984
```

```
Ai-ling Cheng

See Cheng, Ai-ling
```

Original Name **Cross-Reference Card**

Figure 7-6 Cross-Reference for the Name of a Married Woman

```
Moncrief, Gladys A. (Mrs.)

Mrs. Gladys A. Moncrief
427 Oakdale Drive
Lebanon, TN  37087-8837
```

```
Moncrief, Roy (Mrs.)

See Moncrief, Gladys A. (Mrs.)
```

Original Card **Cross-Reference Card**

Figure 7-7 Cross-Reference for Hyphenated Name

```
Armstrong-Jones, Walter

Walter Armstrong-Jones
803 Peachtree Street
Atlanta, GA  30033-1118
```

```
Jones, Walter Armstrong (-)

See Armstrong-Jones, Walter
```

Original Card **Cross-Reference Card**

120 Medical Office Procedures

Figure 7-8 Cross-Reference for a Firm with Multiple Names

```
Adams, George, & Langston, Surveyors

Adams, George & Langston Surveyors
811 Sycamore Street
Cincinnati, OH  45242-9382
```

Original Card

```
George, Langston, & Adams, Surveyors

See Adams, George & Langston, Surveyors
```

Cross-Reference Card

```
Langston, Adams & George, Surveyors

See Adams, Langston, & George, Surveyors
```

Cross-Reference Card

Figure 7-9 Cross-Reference for Single Letters in a Name

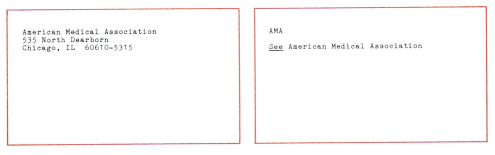

```
American Medical Association
535 North Dearborn
Chicago, IL  60610-5315
```

Original Card

```
AMA

See American Medical Association
```

Cross-Reference Card

Figure 7-10 Cross-Reference for Similar Names*

```
Krause, Walter J.

Walter J. Krause
804 Ecker Drive
Blue Ash, OH  45236-2291
```
Original Card

```
Kraus

See also Crouse, Krass, Krause, Krouse
```
Cross-Reference Card

* A cross reference should be made for each spelling of similar names.

7.24 Alphabetic Filing Procedures

To assure easy retrieval of materials filed by the alphabetic method, follow the steps below:

1. Code the document by underlining the indexing units or by writing the code name in the upper right-hand corner.
2. Cross-reference the document as needed. (See Figures 7-5 through 7-10.)
3. Locate the correct alphabetic guides in the filing system.
4. File the document and any cross-references in the appropriate folders.
5. Retrieve the file folder as needed.

NUMERIC FILING

Numeric filing is a method of filing by number instead of by letter. The numeric method is used in many medical offices to maintain the confidentiality of patient records. A number on a folder tab does not reveal the identity of a patient as easily or as directly as the person's name does. In large medical centers and hospitals with many folders, the numeric method is used to make files easier to retrieve.

7.25 Accession Book or Patient Identification Ledger

The *accession book* or *patient identification ledger* provides a consecutive record of the numbers and names of all patients. When a new patient visits the medical office, the next available number in the accession book is assigned to that patient and the person's name is written beside the number. This number identifies the patient and is written on each paper associated with the patient before the paper is filed. For example, lab reports, case histories, letters, or other documents which refer to the patient are coded with the patient's number.

Numeric procedures can also be used in subject and geographic filing systems. Subjects or geographic names are assigned a number, then a list is maintained which identifies each folder name and its identifying number. Figure 7-11 illustrates an accession book.

Figure 7-11   Accession Book

741 Anne Hill	750
742 Rose Corgan	751
743 Nathan Lee	752
744 Gilda Tudor	753
745 Raymond Reuter	754
746	755
747	756
748	757
749	758

7.26   Alphabetic Card File

An alphabetic card file containing a card for each patient is an essential part of a numeric filing system. Each card lists the patient's full name, address, telephone number, and patient number. Alphabetic cards are stored in a rotary card holder, a card tray, or a card box in alphabetic order according to the patient's last name. When a patient's folder needs to be retrieved, the person's card is located and the patient number is identified from the card. Then the folder matching the number is located in the patient files. A patient alphabetic card is shown in Figure 7-12.

In addition to the patient card file, a separate file is maintained for miscellaneous alphabetic cards. These cards list the names, addresses,

Figure 7-12 Patient Alphabetic Card

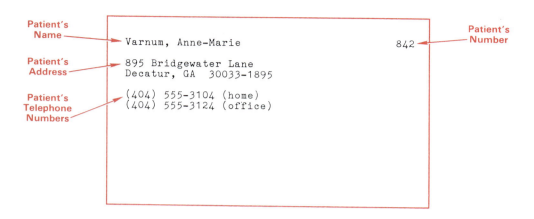

and telephone numbers of ambulance services, hospitals, police, research organizations, professional organizations, suppliers, and other physicians.

7.27 Numeric File Guides and Tabs

Numeric file guides, usually made of cardboard or plastic, break numeric files into manageable sections. Folders may be divided into number groups of 1-99, 100-199, 200-299, for example. Secondary guides are used to subdivide the numbers further and are placed in the second position. The tabs of individual folders are usually shown in third position. Fourth and fifth position folders are available for medical offices requiring them. For purposes of confidentiality, the folder tab usually lists only the patient's number, although in some offices the patient's name is also listed (see Figure 7-13). Folders are stored in ascending order with the smallest number at the front.

Figure 7-13 Numeric Guides and Tabs

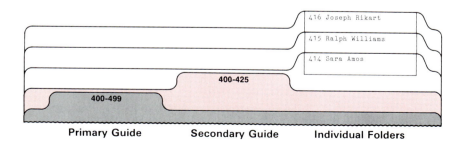

7.28 Miscellaneous Correspondence File

When a numeric system is used for medical records, an alphabetic correspondence file is usually maintained for materials not related to patients. These materials contain general information pertaining to the medical practice, professional organizations, or research. The alphabetic caption on each folder tab identifies the contents of the folder. A separate folder labeled *Miscellaneous* is stored at the back of the file or shelf to hold miscellaneous materials involving fewer than five items about a single subject. When five related items accumulate, a new folder with an appropriate tab caption is prepared and the materials are transferred to this folder. The folder is then merged in alphabetic order with other folders.

7.29 Numeric Filing Procedures

Several steps are necessary to ensure correct numeric filing of materials. When a new patient visits the medical office:

1. Assign the next unused number in the accession book to the patient.
2. Complete an alphabetic card (see Figure 7-12, p. 123).
3. Prepare a file folder listing the patient number on the tab (see Figure 7-13, p. 123).
4. Store the folder in ascending order with the other patient folders.

When a file is to be retrieved:

1. Locate the patient's name in the alphabetic card file and identify the patient's number.
2. Look for the patient's number on the folder tabs of the medical records. Remove the appropriate medical record from the files.
3. Return the folder to the files when there is no further need for it.

SUBJECT FILING

Subject filing is a method of filing by subject titles instead of by individuals' names. Subject titles are used in medical offices to identify diseases, research, treatments, drugs, and other areas of interest to the physician. For example, a physician researching children's diseases may use the captions *diabetes, muscular dystrophy, heart disease,* or others. Letters, memos, research reports, and other items from many different sources are stored in the folders.

The business-related activities of a medical office also lend themselves to subject filing. For example, a medical office may have folder tabs labeled *Medicare, Medicaid, Workers' Compensation, Blue Cross/Blue Shield,* or others. Usually, subject files are stored according to the alphabetic method; however, a number may be assigned to each subject so the folders can be filed by the numeric method.

7.30 Cross-Referencing of Subject Files

Materials filed by subject often need to be cross-referenced because all individuals do not think of them in the same terms. For example, a letter about research on skin disease might be filed by the subject title *Skin Disease* and cross-referenced under the letter writer's name.

7.31 Subject Filing Guides and Tabs

A primary file guide is used to identify the broad subject area of a set of folders. Primary guides are made of heavy cardboard or plastic. Their tabs are visible in the first position of the file drawer or file shelf. Secondary guides, also made of heavy cardboard or plastic, are used to break the broad subject into smaller parts and are placed next to the primary guide. A secondary guide may be subdivided into smaller units with their own guides if additional subcategories are needed. Individual folders should have tab captions located in the last position of the file drawer or file shelf. File folders may be five position, three position, or two position, depending on the number of subdivisions made from the primary subject. Figure 7-14 illustrates a three-position file with a primary guide, a secondary guide, and individual folders.

Figure 7-14   A Three-Position Subject File with Primary Guides, Secondary Guides, and Individual Folders

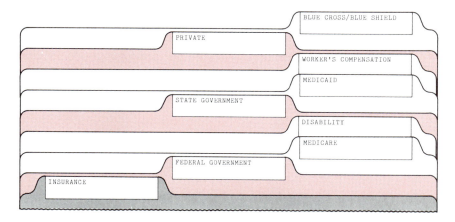

A master sheet listing all subject captions should be available to everyone who uses the filing system to ensure consistent use of captions when filing and retrieving.

7.32 Subject Filing Procedures

1. Prepare a master record of primary and secondary subject captions of file folders (plus the subject number if a numeric system is used).
2. Check each incoming and outgoing document to determine the subject title under which the document should be filed.
3. Code the document by underlining the subject caption or writing the subject caption in the upper right-hand corner.
4. Make a cross-reference sheet when a document might be identified by more than one subject.
5. Store the document and the cross-reference sheet in the correct folders.
6. Store the folder in alphabetic order in the subject file.
7. Retrieve as needed.

GEOGRAPHIC FILING

Geographic filing is a method of filing by geographic area instead of by a person's name or by a subject. Often geographic and subject methods are used together. While geographic files are not found in most medical offices, they are useful in medical research centers to identify regions of the country in which research is conducted. For example, the geographic method might be used to identify states or regions in which research into allergies is being conducted. Geographic materials may be stored by the alphabetic or numeric methods.

7.33 Cross-Referencing of Geographic Filing Systems

Cross-referencing is important to the geographic system since all individuals who use the materials may not think in terms of the same geographic areas. A cross-reference should be made for each piece of material which might be difficult to locate (see Section 7.23).

7.34 Geographic Filing Guides and Tabs

The primary guide in a geographic system is made of heavy cardboard or plastic and identifies a broad geographic area. Secondary guides are used to break geographic areas into smaller components.

Folder captions identify an additional geographic breakdown or a subject area related to the region shown in the primary and secondary guides. Figure 7-15 illustrates a geographic file.

Figure 7-15   Geographic File with Primary and Secondary Guides

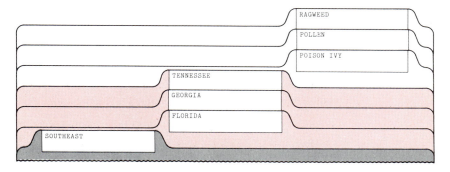

7.35   Geographic Filing Procedures

1. Prepare a master record of the geographic tab captions.

2. Check each incoming and outgoing document to determine the geographic code under which the document should be filed.

3. Code the document by underlining the geographic tab caption or writing the caption in the upper right-hand corner.

4. Make a cross-reference sheet when a document might be identified in more than one way.

5. File the document and the cross-reference sheet in the correct folders.

6. Store the folder in alphabetic order in the geographic files.

7. Retrieve as needed.

COLOR IN MEDICAL FILING SYSTEMS

Color can be used effectively and attractively in the medical office to ensure quick, accurate filing and retrieval of patient records. Commercial filing systems that combine letters of the alphabet with color can be customized for any medical office.

7.36   Open-Shelf Filing Cabinets with Colored Folder Tabs

The most common type of filing cabinet used in a medical office is an open-shelf cabinet. File folders with side tabs, instead of the traditional top tabs, are stored on stationary or pull-out open shelves. The folder tabs, which extend beyond the side of file folders, show the caption or name of the folder. Three-, four-, or five-position folders, available from medical office supply firms, are popular in most medical offices. The number of tab positions is determined by the filing method used. Tab position one refers to the position at the top of the folder and is followed by the remaining positions down the edge of the folder.

7.37 Color Coding Patient Names

In the TAB AlphaCode system, which is representative of color coding systems used in medical offices, the following formula is used for labeling folders (see Figure 7-16):

Position One - Primary guides dividing the alphabet
Extension to Position One - Last year patient was seen
Position Two - Label with patient's full name, last name first
Positions Three, Four, Five - First three letters of the patient's last name

Figure 7-16 File with Color Codes

```
         D
              1983    Cram, Roberta L.        C  C  C    R
              1984    Cermak, Charles M.      C  C  C    E
              1984    Carlton, Janice K.      C  C  C    A
              1985    Caton, Bruce G.         C  A  A    E
         C
```

When folders are filed correctly on a shelf, large patterns of color blocks are created. An out-of-place file breaks the color pattern, making misfiles easy to detect. In the name *Caton,* for example, the *C* is represented by orange and the *a* by brown. Folders for other patients whose last names start with *Ca* also show orange and brown in positions three and four. If a folder showing orange and green in third and fourth positions (representing *Ce*) is filed incorrectly with the *Ca* folders, it is readily visible because the color pattern is interrupted.

Rolls of adhesive-backed color-coded labels are available from medical office suppliers. Manufacturers of filing equipment and supplies can also develop computer-generated color codes based on the patient list of an individual medical office.

7.38 Color Coding Patient Numbers

In the same way that different colors represent letters of the alphabet, different colors represent the numbers zero through nine. The patients' numbers are color coded in positions one through five, creating large blocks of color when folders are filed correctly. For example, in the TAB CompuColor numeric filing system, one is represented by purple, six by blue, eight by rose, nine by brown, and zero by pink. The patient number 16890 is represented by the following color codes in positions one through five: purple, blue, rose, brown, and pink. Color patterns are formed by the correct filing of folders. Any folder stored out of sequence will be visible immediately.

7.39 Using Color to Identify Patients for Different Physicians

When several physicians share an office, it is easy to separate folders by using a different color stripe across the name label in position two to represent the primary care physician. For example, a green stripe may represent all of the patients for Physician No. 1. Only patients assigned to Physician No. 1 will have their folders coded with a green stripe. Patients under the care of Physicians No. 2 and 3 are represented by other color stripes.

7.40 Out Guides

When a folder is taken from the files, an *out guide* is placed in the folder's original position. A charge-out slip showing who has the folder and when it will be returned is placed in a side pocket. A second side pocket can be used to store material which would have been added to the removed folder. Color-coded out guides, which make removed folders easier to recognize, can be purchased from medical office suppliers.

CREATING A PATIENT FILE

A *patient file* consists of all information which a medical office maintains about an individual patient. When the medical office keeps a traditional paper file, it consists of three elements: (1) the medical record, which contains medical information about the patient (see Chapter 5); (2) the ledger card, which gives billing information about the patient's account (see Chapter 11); and (3) the alphabetic card, which is a quick reference for the patient's telephone number, address, and patient number (see Section 7.26). (The alphabetic card is optional in offices which do not use a numeric filing system.) When the file is computerized, patient information is filed automatically according to the patient's name or the patient's number. In many offices the ledger card and a patient list are computerized, while the medical record is maintained in the traditional manner.

The patient file should not be confused with the medical record, which is sometimes called the patient record. The medical record is only one element of a complete patient file.

7.41 Instructions for Creating a Patient File

A patient file is created during the initial visit of each new patient. Ask the patient to arrive a few minutes early to allow time for gathering the necessary information.

Follow these steps to create a patient file:

1. Ask the new patient to complete a Patient Information Form (see Section 5.1) and a Patient Questionnaire (see Section 5.2). Attach the forms to a clipboard. Give the patient a pen or pencil with which to complete the forms. You may need to assist the patient in filling out the form.

2. If a numeric filing system is used, assign the new patient the next unused number in the accession book.

3. Type a label showing the patient's name or number, and birthdate. Attach the label to a blank file folder. Add color-coding labels (see Sections 7.36-7.40).

4. Staple or clip the patient information form to the left side of the file folder.

5. Bind the patient's history form to the inside, right side of the folder.

6. Type the heading on a ledger card showing the patient's name, address, and patient number, if used.

7. File the ledger card in alphabetic order in the ledger card file.

8. Type an alphabetic card showing the patient's name, address, patient number, if used, and telephone number.

9. File the alphabetic card in correct order in the alphabetic card file.

10. After the patient has seen the doctor, file the medical record in correct alphabetic or numeric order in the medical records file.

7.42 Creating a Patient File: Computerized Records

A computer can be used to create patient files, including the medical record, the ledger card, and the alphabetic card. Once information is entered into the computer, a variety of documents can be produced automatically, including insurance forms, monthly statements, alphabetic or numeric patient lists, deposit slips, and financial records (see Chapter 14).

8

Scheduling

Efficient management of a medical office depends on the proper scheduling of appointments for patients and other visitors. If appointments are scheduled too close together, patients must wait to see the physician. If appointments are scheduled too far apart, valuable time is lost.

THE APPOINTMENT BOOK

8.1 Description of the Appointment Book

The appointment book is the daily planning guide for physicians and their staffs. It shows (1) the names of the patients to be seen each day, (2) the time of each patient's appointment, and (3) a brief reason for each patient's visit. The patient's phone number should also be listed in case the appointment needs to be rescheduled.

Appointment books are available in several styles, for both single and group practices. They are divided by the days of the week, with the day divided into segments for easy scheduling. Figure 8-1 illustrates a single practice appointment book. Figure 8-2 illustrates a group practice appointment book.

8.2 Routine Appointments

Patient appointments vary in length depending on the reason for the appointment and the doctor's specialty. All medical offices follow a formula for scheduling appointments, and these formulas are fairly standard among practices of the same specialty. A typical scheduling formula for a general practice is shown below:

New patients	30 minutes
Patients for consultation	45 minutes
Patients requiring complete physical examinations	45 minutes
All other patients (minor illnesses, routine checkups)	15 minutes

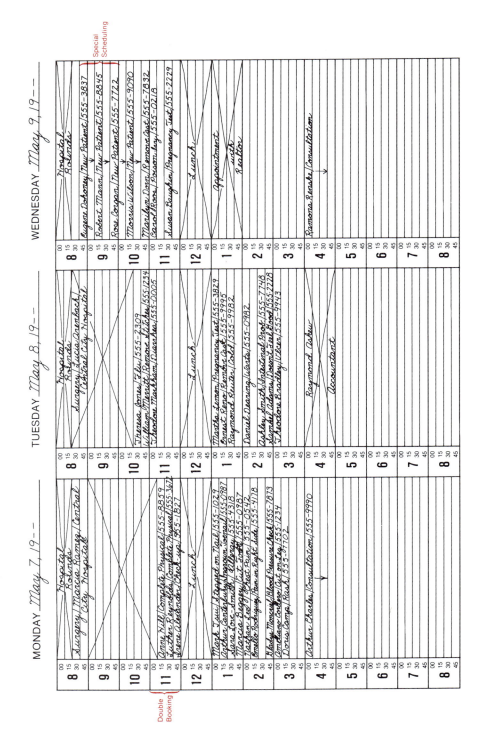

Figure 8-1 Appointment Book Page from a Single Practice

Chapter 8—Scheduling 133

Figure 8-2 Appointment Book Page from a Group Practice

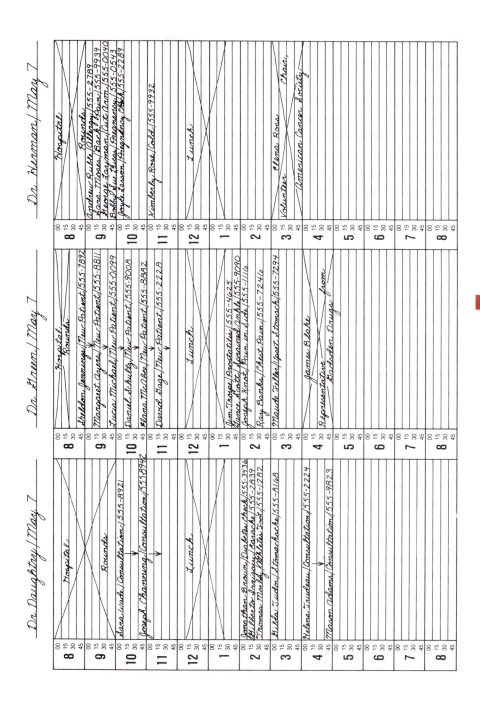

In some medical offices, time is left open once or twice a day so the doctor may see patients who are sick but do not have appointments. The physician's specialty dictates whether time should be set aside, and if so, how much. A pediatrician, for example, is likely to need more unscheduled patient time than a urologist. Refer to Figure 8-1 for examples of patient scheduling.

8.3 Emergencies

When a medical emergency occurs, the injured or sick patient must see the physician immediately. Appointments for other patients are rearranged to accommodate the emergency patient. If you expect the emergency to be resolved in a short time, tell waiting patients of the emergency and assure them that the delay will be short. If the emergency requires a large block of time, waiting patients may be asked to come back later in the day. You should call patients who have not arrived at the office to reschedule their appointments for later the same day or for another day convenient to the patient.

8.4 Recording Appointments

Routine Appointments. The first and last names of each patient are written neatly in the appointment book beside the time of the appointment. A slash mark or dash follows the name, then the patient's complaint or a brief reason for the visit is listed. The patient's telephone number should also be shown. The words *new patient* are written beside the names of all first-time patients. Figure 8-3 illustrates the notation for a routine appointment.

Figure 8-3 Record of Routine Appointment

10	00	Louise Abernathy / Chest Pain / 555-1094
	15	Theresa Mc Farland / Sinus / 555-2084
	30	
	45	

Lengthy Appointments. When an appointment requires more than 15 minutes, ditto marks or an arrow are written in the appointment book to show that additional time periods are needed. The ditto marks or arrows alert everyone using the appointment book that the designated times cannot be scheduled. Figure 8-4 illustrates the notation which is made for a lengthy appointment.

Figure 8-4 Record of Lengthy Appointment

11	00	Lukina Athota / Consultation / 555-0261
	15	″
	30	″
	45	

When the Doctor Is Unavailable. A large "X" is drawn in pencil through all time periods when the physician will not be available for appointments, and a brief explanation is given. Examples of such occasions include (1) morning and evening hospital rounds, (2) lunch time, (3) vacations, (4) business appointments, (5) personal appointments, (6) conventions, and (7) out-of-town trips. Figure 8-5 illustrates the notation that is made when the physician will be unavailable to see patients.

Figure 8-5 Notation to Show Unavailability of Physician

8.5 Double Booking

Double booking is a scheduling system which allows more than one patient to have an appointment for a particular time. The success of double booking depends on the proper combination of patient complaints. A patient having a cut rechecked and a patient having a strep throat rechecked might successfully be booked at the same time because both of their appointments will be brief. A new patient and an established patient may be scheduled for the same time, allowing the established patient to see the doctor while the new patient completes routine forms. Double booking involves risk since someone always has to wait. A medical practice may lose the goodwill of its patients if they must always wait to see the doctor. In a group practice, patients seeing different doctors may be routinely scheduled for the same time.

8.6 Special Scheduling

Special scheduling is used effectively for certain categories of patients. All patients requiring complete physical examinations, for example, may be scheduled for early in the morning or late in the afternoon. Nurses can complete routine tests while the physician makes hospital rounds. Then the patients are ready for further examination and treatment when the physician arrives. Other patients who can be scheduled effectively for special times include individuals requiring X rays or injections, new patients, and maternity patients. The doctor's specialty dictates the occasions when special scheduling is worthwhile.

136   Medical Office Procedures

8.7 The Daily List of Appointments

The daily list of appointments shows the names of all patients to be seen in one day, the patient's complaint or reason for the visit, and the time of each appointment. This daily list is usually typed on plain paper and is copied for the physician, the nurse, the medical assistant, the medical secretary, and others who work with patients. In some offices, the daily page from the appointment book is copied and distributed, eliminating the need for typing the list. The daily list may be prepared at the end of the preceding workday or it may be prepared first thing each morning.

As each medical office employee attends to a patient, a check mark (√) is made beside the patient's name to show which patients have been seen. The receptionist checks off the name after each patient's medical record has been prepared for the nurse; the nurse checks off the name after routine tests have been administered; and the physician checks off the name following examination and treatment. Figure 8-6 illustrates a daily list of appointments.

8.8 Rescheduling Appointments

When either the patient or the physician cannot keep an appointment, it is rescheduled for the first available opening. This is especially important when the appointment is rescheduled at the physician's request.

When an appointment is rescheduled, the appointment book should be corrected by drawing a line through the patient's name and placing a check mark following the name to indicate the rescheduling.

8.9 Cancelling Appointments

While patients are discouraged from cancelling appointments, physicians prefer cancelled appointments to no-show appointments. When an appointment is cancelled, draw a line through the name to indicate the cancellation. The time slot becomes available for another patient. Ask when the patient would like to schedule another appointment, then try to schedule the patient accordingly. If the preferred date and time are already scheduled, suggest an alternative. The cancelled appointment should be noted in the patient's medical record.

8.10 Missed Appointments

Sometimes patients miss appointments without calling to cancel. This wastes time and costs the medical practice money. When a patient misses an appointment, draw a line through the name and write *missed*

Figure 8-6 Daily List of Appointments

```
                    JOHN H. SPARKS, M.D.


                    Daily List of Appointments
                          May 7, 19--

      7:30          Hospital Rounds
      8:30          SURGERY/Marcia Ramez/Central City Hospital
      8:45                      "
      9:00                      "
      9:15                      "
      9:30                      "
      9:45                      "
     10:00                      "
     10:15                      "
     10:30                      "
     10:45                      "
     11:00                      "
     11:15          Anne Hill/Complete physical exam      ⎫ Double
     11:30          Luther Reynolds/Complete physical exam⎬ booking;
     11:45          Irene Alexander/Check-up              ⎭ both
     12:00          Lunch                                   require
                                                            45 minutes
      1:00          Mark Tsui/Stepped on nail
      1:15          Arthur Canterbury/Ingrown toenail
      1:30          Sara Love-Smith/Allergy
      1:45          Marcia Beggey/Cut foot
      2:00          Nathan Lee/Chest pain
      2:15          Emelio Rodriguez/Pain in right side
      2:30
      2:45          Gladys Moncrief/Blood pressure check
      3:00          Ameliano Cordero/Cut on leg
      3:15          Doris Camp/Rash
      3:30
      3:45
      4:00          Arthur Charles/Consultation
      4:15                      "
      4:30                      "
```

or *no show*. Then send a reminder of the missed appointment to the patient's home. Note the *no show* in the patient's medical record.

Some physicians charge for missed appointments. When a patient's account is to be charged, add a line to the appointment reminder card stating this policy. Alert the bookkeeper to charge the patient for the missed appointment. Figure 8-7 illustrates a card reminding the patient of a missed appointment.

Figure 8-7 Reminder of Missed Appointment

DID YOU FORGET...
your appointment on _May 4_
at _10:00_ (a.m.)/p.m.?

Your account has been charged. Please let us know if you would like to reschedule your appointment.

John H. Sparks, M.D.
8504 Capricorn Drive
Atlanta, GA 30033-7775
555-0078

8.11 Nonpatient Appointments

Nonpatient visitors to the medical office may include the physician's accountant or stockbroker, other physicians, certain pharmaceutical or equipment representatives, and family members. These visitors are generally scheduled during nonpatient hours, such as early morning or late afternoon. A visiting physician or the doctor's family, however, is allowed to see the doctor as soon as possible, usually between patients. Check with your physician-employer to determine which visitors are to be given appointments, then screen visitors carefully to make certain that only those whom the physician wishes to see are granted appointments.

8.12 Walk-in Patients Without Appointments

Although most physicians in private practice discourage nonemergency patients from coming to the medical office without an appointment, this sometimes happens. If time is available for a walk-in patient, the physician will see the person. If no time is available, try to schedule an appointment at an open time. Emergency patients, of course, should see the physician immediately.

8.13 Arranging Follow-up Appointments

When a patient needs to return for follow-up treatment or for a checkup, the physician tells the nurse or indicates the follow-up on the patient's superbill (charge slip). Appointments, except for those needed more than six months in the future, are scheduled at the time of the initial visit. If several follow-up appointments are needed, as in the case of a maternity patient, they may all be scheduled at the time of the initial visit. Give the patient a card showing the date and time of the next appointment. Figure 8-8 illustrates a follow-up reminder card.

Figure 8-8 Card Showing Follow-up Appointment

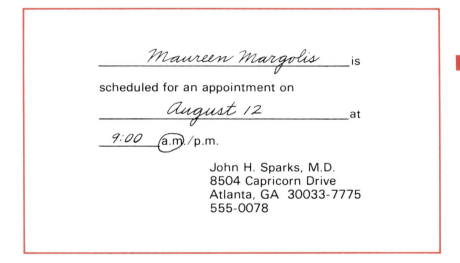

8.14 Follow-up in Several Months

Many patients routinely see their physician every six months or every year for a checkup. When the appointment is for the distant future, it is not always feasible to schedule it at the time of the initial visit. Instead, a tickler file is maintained for follow-up appointments.

The tickler file contains cards showing the names and addresses of patients needing follow-up appointments. The cards are filed behind monthly dividers according to month and date. Once a month the follow-up cards are retrieved and mailed to patients needing follow-up appointments within the next two months.

Preprinted reminder cards are available from medical forms suppliers. After the patient addresses the cards at the initial visit, they are stored in the tickler file. At retrieval time, they are stamped and mailed. Figure 8-9 illustrates a preprinted follow-up reminder card.

Figure 8-9   Preprinted Follow-up Reminder Card

> It is time for your *annual*
> checkup. Please call the office so that
> we may schedule an appointment for you.
>
> John H. Sparks, M.D.
> 8504 Capricorn Drive
> Atlanta, GA 30033-7775
> 555-0078

SCHEDULING PATIENTS FOR THE HOSPITAL AND OTHER MEDICAL FACILITIES

8.15   Nonsurgical Treatment in the Hospital

When a patient is to be admitted to a hospital, the physician gives admitting information to a nurse or another medical office employee who contacts the hospital admitting office. The information which the admitting office requires includes the patient's name, address, and phone number; the names of the admitting physician and the assisting physician; the diagnosis; the medications required; the preferred admittance date; and the type of room. The admitting office schedules an admittance date based on the availability of a room or bed.

8.16   Surgery in the Hospital

When surgery is to be performed in the hospital, the medical office employee books the patient for an operating room. The operating room scheduling clerk needs the following information: the type of surgery, the approximate amount of time required, names of all physicians who will be operating or assisting, and the preferred time. After arrangements are complete, the medical office employee relays to the patient all necessary information concerning the surgery and hospitalization.

When another physician is needed for assisting or consulting in the operating room, the medical office employee makes the arrangements with the consulting physician's secretary before scheduling the operating room.

8.17 Emergency Hospital Treatment

Sometimes patients call or come to the medical office when they need emergency hospital treatment. When this happens, ask the physician how the situation should be handled. If the physician is not in the office, give the patient directions to the hospital and ask the person to go immediately to the emergency room. If the patient has no means of transportation or is too ill to drive, call the life squad and arrange to have the patient taken to the hospital. Then call the hospital emergency room to notify the staff that the patient will be arriving. Provide as much information as you can regarding the patient's symptoms. Locate the physician and tell the doctor that the emergency patient is on the way to the hospital.

8.18 Scheduling for Therapy, X ray, Tests, and Other Medical Services

Patients frequently require medical services which must be performed outside the physician's office, either by another physician, by a laboratory, or by a specialty medical service. These patients may schedule their own appointments, or the medical office employee may make the arrangements for them. If you make the appointment, call while the patient is in the office, and ask for a time convenient to the patient. Provide the patient's name and the physician's name, plus information regarding the service to be performed or the type of test to be given. After arrangements are complete, give the patient a card which shows the time, date, and place of the appointment.

Sometimes physicians refer their patients to the hospital for outpatient care, which can include laboratory services and minor surgery. The medical office employee's responsibility is to provide the hospital with information about the patient and the services to be performed and to provide the patient with the date and time of surgery plus other details relevant to the outpatient care.

9

Travel Arrangements

Since medical research and experimentation is conducted all over the world, communication is a vital link in the medical field. While much information is communicated through medical journals and other correspondence, a considerable amount of communication and learning takes place at medical conferences and during visits to other medical facilities. The medical office employee is often involved in making the complex arrangements for this important travel.

It will be helpful for you to find one or more travel agents to assist you with the task of making travel arrangements. Using a travel agent will not increase the cost of travel because commissions are paid to a travel agent by the airlines, hotels, and car rental agencies. Many travel agents lease computer terminals from one of the major airlines. The terminals keep them up-to-date on the latest fare discounts and flight schedules for all airlines, and give them information on package travel plans, hotel availability, and special events in various locations. Travel arrangements can be made by telephone when credit card signatures are kept on file with the travel agent. If you repeatedly use the services of a specific travel agent, an account can usually be set up for your office, and the travel agent will send one invoice for the costs of all travel.

9.1 Air Transportation

Most travel will involve air transportation, since flying is a time-saving way to travel. One good source of flight information is the *Official Airline Guide (OAG)*. The *OAG* lists all airline carriers serving a particular area, as well as regular flights offered. When making reservations, however, confirm *OAG* flight information and ask for cancellations, new flights, and special fare packages. Before airline reservations can be made, you will need the following information from the medical personnel preparing to travel:

Destination.   What cities, states, and countries are involved?

Dates and Times Preferred. On what date do the travelers want to arrive in each city, state, country; and on what date do they want to depart? Within a three-hour time block, when would they prefer to leave (or when would they prefer to arrive at the destination)?

Airline Preference. Is there a preferred airline? Some medical personnel will collect frequent flyer bonus miles from airlines that have such programs and may wish to fly only on those airlines. Such plans will bring cost reductions for future flights, or free flights following the accumulation of a required number of miles with the participating airline.

Cost Versus Convenience. It is helpful to know which is more important: cost or convenience. Would the medical traveler prefer first-class travel? What about changing travel dates to save dollars? Travel during weekdays and nonholiday times will often be less expensive. Making reservations at least a month in advance and prepaying tickets can also reduce travel costs. If time is important, will the traveler fly first class if that is all that is available? Higher priced first-class fares provide personal service, additional seating space, free drinks, improved meal service and choices, and free movies (if offered on the flight). Since additional costs for first-class travel vary, check with your travel agent or airline travel desk for accurate information.

Determine Restrictions. It is important that you understand the restrictions that apply to the airline reservations you make. Reservations for some fares cannot be changed without adding to the cost of the tickets. The traveler may be restricted to certain days of the week, or a certain minimum or maximum stay may be required to guarantee a discount fare. Determine the requirements for cancelling reservations. Airline tickets should be safeguarded as carefully as cash. Unused tickets should be returned promptly to the place of purchase for proper credit. Lost or stolen tickets should be reported immediately to the airline. The traveler should be prepared to pay for replacement airline tickets, and wait 30-90 days for a refund if lost or stolen tickets are not used. If the traveler misses a flight because of the airline (late connecting flight), the airline should provide alternative air travel at no additional charge. When a missed flight is the traveler's responsibility, however, new flight arrangements may result in additional costs. Make a list of any restrictions that apply and give them to the medical traveler along with the airline tickets.

9.2 Ground Transportation

Some medical personnel prefer not to fly. In such cases, travel arrangements are made for train or bus transportation in much the same way airline arrangements are made.

Sometimes medical personnel may want to drive their own automobiles to their destinations. In such cases, it is helpful to use the services of a travel club, such as the American Automobile Association (AAA). Such travel clubs can help by providing road maps with the best routes highlighted, information about cities along the way, recommendations for lodgings, and discounts on some services.

Local transportation is usually required for the airline, train, or bus traveler. Ask the travel agent or reservation personnel about transportation available between the airport, train station, or bus terminal and the hotel (taxis, limousines, courtesy buses, city buses). These options should be listed for the traveler. Find out if the medical traveler will require a rental car. Many airlines offer special discounts on car rentals when airline tickets are purchased. Travel agents can recommend special package rates for car rentals combined with airline and hotel accommodations. Of course, car rental agencies can also be contacted directly. Ask about special discounts or package pricing.

9.3 Hotel Reservations

When making hotel reservations, it is important to know where the medical traveler will need to be in the city visited. Medical conferences or conventions will designate a headquarters hotel. If a convention center or medical complex is to be used for meetings, check to see which hotels are located within walking distance of the complex. You can get brochures describing the medical conference and the planned activities from the sponsoring organization, your travel agent, or from the Chamber of Commerce in the city to be visited. When making reservations with the hotel (or through the travel agent), ask if there are special discount rates available at the hotel for this particular medical conference. You need to know if the medical traveler will require a single or double room, and any other special arrangements that should be made with the hotel. If you must arrange a meeting or luncheon hosted by your medical traveler, speak with the hotel sales or catering office. They will be able to help you with all the details as well as offer expert advice.

Some hotels have 800 numbers, which make calls for reservations and information toll free. Another way to avoid the inconvenience of long-distance calling is to call local hotels that are part of a chain. They can often make reservations for hotels in other cities that are part of the same chain.

Ask for the name of a contact person at the hotel and for a confirmation number when making reservations, or for a cancellation number for making cancellations. Knowing a name and number will make things easier if you later have to change the arrangements. Special requests for oceanview rooms, ground or upper floor rooms, or rooms near stairs or elevators should be made when making reservations and confirmed at check-in. Be prepared to provide a credit card number for guaranteed (prepaid) reservations. Guaranteed reservations are advisable if the traveler plans to arrive late in the evening. You will also need to know how long the traveler plans to stay at the hotel.

Obtain information on check-in and check-out times. When hotel reservations are final, the hotel will send you a written confirmation.

9.4 Traveler's Checks

Encourage the traveler to use traveler's checks rather than carry large amounts of cash. Traveler's checks can be replaced if lost or stolen.

9.5 Prepare an Itinerary

Prepare a typed itinerary so that the traveler will have a convenient record of all of the arrangements you have made (see Figure 9-1). Since all arrival times are indicated in local time, indicate to the traveler where time zones have been crossed. Prepare at least three copies of the itinerary; one for the traveler, one for the office, and one for the traveler's family. Keep a record of the numbers of all flights, tickets, credit cards used, and traveler's checks in case the traveler's package (see Section 9.7) is lost or stolen.

9.6 Expense Account Forms

Obtain a copy of a blank travel expense form used by your medical office. Include this form in the travel package (see Section 9.7) you are preparing for the medical traveler. The traveler can then record expenses and attach necessary receipts while travel is in progress and details are easily remembered. Upon return to the medical office, a final report can quickly be typed and submitted for reimbursement. Records required for reimbursement may include airline ticket stubs; hotel bills; and restaurant, taxi, and rental car receipts.

9.7 The Traveler's Package

Within a file folder or large envelope, place the following items:

1. Airline, train, or bus tickets (including information regarding any restrictions)

Figure 9-1 Itinerary

```
                          ITINERARY
                       Dr. Lenore Berger

NATIONAL CONFERENCE ON SPORTS MEDICINE
Chicago, Illinois                              August 2-7, 19--
----------------------------------------------------------------

Leave      Miami      Sunday, August 1    3:15 p.m.
                                          Omega Airline
                                          Flight #84 to Atlanta
                                          (arrive 4:03 p.m.)

                      NOTE:  Present Frequent Flyer Coupon with
                             ticket to agent at gate

Leave      Atlanta    Sunday, August 1    4:55 p.m.
                                          Omega Airline
                                          Flight #73 to Chicago

                      NOTE:  Present Frequent Flyer Coupon with
                             ticket to agent at gate

Arrive     Chicago    Sunday, August 1    5:30 p.m. (Chicago time)
----------------------------------------------------------------
```

Hotel accommodations at the Barony Hotel on Jefferson Avenue, confirmation attached. Room will be ready when you arrive. This is the headquarters hotel for the conference.

NATIONAL CONFERENCE ON SPORTS MEDICINE begins on Monday, August 2, with registration at 8:30 a.m. (See conference material enclosed.)

Note: Dr. Kenneth Springer would like to meet you for lunch on Tuesday, August 3. He will call you in your room sometime Sunday evening following your arrival.

```
----------------------------------------------------------------

Note:  Hotel check-out time -- 1:00 p.m.

Leave      Chicago    Saturday, August 7   3:00 p.m. (Chicago time)
                                           Omega Airline
                                           Flight #87

                      NOTE:  Present Frequent Flyer Coupon with
                             ticket to agent at gate

Arrive     Miami      Saturday, August 7   7:01 p.m. (Miami time)
                             WELCOME HOME!
```

2. The traveler's itinerary

3. Ground transportation options

4. Information regarding the medical conference/meeting and any appointments the traveler may have

5. Hotel confirmation

6. Car rental confirmation

7. Blank travel expense form

8. Extra business cards

9. Pad of paper and a pen or pencil

10. Maps of the city and any other information you have been able to obtain regarding the city to be visited

9.8   Foreign Travel

Requirements for travel abroad are more complex than those for domestic travel. Check with a travel agent or airline regarding requirements for a current passport and entry visa. Allow three to six weeks to obtain a new passport. Time requirements for visas vary according to the country. Your travel agent or the local consulate of the country to be visited will be of great assistance in obtaining information regarding visas, transportation, currency exchange, hotel accommodations, and other travel needs. Before leaving, it is recommended that at least a small amount of cash be exchanged for the currency of the country to be visited. Transportation to the hotel and tips to baggage handlers can then be covered in the local currency before exchanging larger amounts of cash at a local bank or hotel.

10

Health Insurance

Most people have some form of health care insurance which pays a portion or all of the expenses of a treated illness or injury. It may be group insurance, individual insurance, government-sponsored insurance, or membership in a health plan or health maintenance organization. Benefits vary widely from policy to policy. Some insurance policies cover all the expenses of an illness or injury while others provide limited benefits. Generally the amount of coverage rises in proportion to the size of the premium. The patient is ultimately responsible for the payment of the account and must pay any difference between the charges of the physician or other medical provider and the insurance coverage.

When a patient is treated at a medical facility, either the patient or the medical facility files a claim with the insurance carrier for payment of the physician's fees, surgery fees, hospital care, and other related medical services. The carrier's claim department reviews the claim to determine whether the patient's policy covers the services performed. If the patient is covered, the carrier mails a check directly to the physician or to the patient. Some physicians require payment at the time of their service. In such cases the patient pays the physician, then files a claim for reimbursement.

Since the claim process can be lengthy, clear documentation of each illness or medical service is important. The insurance claim form must be completed fully and accurately. If the claim is questioned because the form is incomplete or unclear, payment will be delayed until the insurance carrier is provided with the information it needs. Since delayed payments are costly to a medical practice, it is your responsibility to eliminate them when possible.

TYPES OF HEALTH CARE COVERAGE

Since many patients depend on health care coverage to pay for all or a portion of their medical expenses, it is important for you to determine what coverage the patient carries. The best way to obtain this information is to provide space on the patient information form for the names of all insurance carriers and the numbers of each policy (see Section 5.1, Figure 5-1). You can also ask to see the patient's insurance identification card which is issued with the policy. This card shows the name of the carrier and the policy number.

10.1 Health Insurance

Group Health Insurance. Group health insurance is designed for a group of people who have something in common that makes them insurable. They may work for the same company, belong to the same professional organization, or be a member of the same profession. Each person is insured under one group policy. All members of the group receive the same coverage and pay the same premium. Companies frequently offer group insurance to employees at a reduced cost or at no cost as an employee benefit.

While group health insurance differs from company to company, the coverage usually pays for physicians' services, hospital care, surgery, and related services for the policyholder and the policyholder's dependents. Health insurance is divided into two categories—basic health insurance and major medical insurance. *Basic health insurance* pays for basic medical services and limits the amount the insurance company pays for any one illness. For example, the number of days of hospitalization paid for any one illness is set at the time the policy is purchased. *Major medical insurance* pays for additional medical services, including extra days of hospital care not covered by basic insurance. A person with both basic health insurance and major medical insurance is covered for most medical expenses.

Individual Health Insurance. Individual health insurance, or private health insurance, is tailored to the needs of an individual and the individual's dependents. The benefits of individual policies vary, but they are similar to the benefits of group insurance policies. Individual coverage is usually more expensive than group coverage.

10.2 Blue Cross/Blue Shield

Blue Cross and Blue Shield is a nonprofit organization which provides prepaid health care coverage to subscribers in designated geographic areas. Several different Blue Cross/Blue Shield plans exist around the country. Each plan develops and administers its own benefits package. Blue Shield plans provide coverage for physicians' services and surgery; Blue Cross plans provide coverage for hospital expenses. Many people subscribe to both plans.

Blue Cross/Blue Shield plans usually cover groups of people. For example, all the employees of a single company may be covered as group members of a Blue Cross/Blue Shield plan. Blue Cross/Blue Shield plans are available for individual subscribers also. Some members convert to individual plans when they leave a company's group plan.

10.3 Health Maintenance Organizations (HMOs)

Health maintenance organizations offer prepaid medical services to members. The emphasis of HMOs is on wellness rather than illness. Health maintenance organizations may be operated by an employer, a medical school, a labor union, or some other recognized group. Members pay a fixed premium in advance in return for the medical care they may need. The premium is paid even if the medical service is not used. Employers often offer membership in a health maintenance organization as a benefit of employment with the company.

The two types of health maintenance organizations are the *closed panel* and the *open panel*. In the closed panel organization, a group of salaried physicians use facilities owned by the organization. In the open panel organization, the organization contracts with physicians and hospitals to offer services on a fixed-fee basis. When an HMO member develops a medical problem, the person goes to the location and physician(s) named in the plan. While HMO members lose the opportunity to choose a medical provider, many people seek more medical care than they otherwise would, since the care is paid for in advance.

HMO plans vary in the same way that insurance policies vary. The benefits offered by one HMO plan are not necessarily the same as those offered by another.

10.4 Preferred Provider Organization (PPO)

An employer or other group may sign a contract with a health provider, such as a medical center or hospital, to provide medical services for all employees or members of the group. A predetermined volume of business is guaranteed in return for discounts on services.

10.5 Medicare

Medicare is a health insurance program of the federal government's Social Security Administration. It is designed to provide health care for individuals 65 or older and to disabled people under 65. Medicare consists of two parts: hospital insurance and medical insurance. Hospital insurance pays for most but not all hospital care and related expenses. The rates paid by Medicare for hospital charges are determined by diagnosis related groups (DRGs) (see Section 10.10). Medicare medical insurance pays 80 percent of reasonable physicians' fees and related medical charges minus a deductible amount. In each state, an administering group is named to process the Medicare claims. The Equitable Life Assurance Society, Aetna Life & Casualty, and Nationwide Insurance are examples of state administrators. To determine the name of the Medicare administrator in your state, call your local Medicare office.

Medicare recipients are issued cards showing whether they have only hospital benefits or hospital and medical benefits. The card also shows the Medicare identification number. When you are working with a Medicare patient, ask for the patient's card in order to determine coverage. Medicare accepts the Universal Health Insurance Claim Form shown in Section 10.13, Figure 10-4.

10.6 Medicaid

Medicaid is a financial assistance program developed jointly by the federal government and the states to provide health care for needy people. Benefits are similar to other insurance programs, though benefits differ from state to state. Medicaid generally pays the deductible amount under Medicare and the 20 percent not covered by Medicare medical insurance. You should check with your local Medicaid office to determine what Medicaid benefits are paid in your state.

Medicaid claim forms are filed with the state administering agent. Time limits for filing claims vary from state to state. Be sure to determine the deadline for filing claims; late claims may be rejected by the Medicaid administrator. Since Medicaid claim forms differ from state to state, no form is shown here. The Universal Health Care Claim Form shown in Section 10.13, Figure 10-4, is accepted in many states.

10.7 CHAMPUS/CHAMPVA

CHAMPUS is the Civilian Health and Medical Program of the Uniformed Services (Army, Navy, Air Force, for example). This program covers medical care that is not directly related to the service for uniformed services personnel and their families. While most uniformed services families obtain their medical care from government facilities, they are paid CHAMPUS benefits if they are referred to a private physician. The individual or agency providing medical service must be authorized by CHAMPUS.

Dependents who prefer to be treated by a civilian medical facility can receive care by providing a nonavailability statement issued by the commander of the military hospital. This statement should be attached to the CHAMPUS claim reporting form. CHAMPUS Form 500 or the Universal Health Insurance Claim Form, shown in Figure 10-4, may be used for filing claims.

CHAMPVA refers to the Civilian Health and Medical Program of the Veterans Administration and is similar to CHAMPUS. Individuals covered are (1) dependents of totally disabled veterans whose disabilities are service related and (2) surviving dependents of veterans who have died from service-related disabilities. CHAMPUS Form 500 may be used for filing claims.

10.8 Workers' Compensation

Workers' compensation is an income maintenance and health care insurance program established by law in each state to cover occupational diseases and work-related injury or death. Excluded from the workers' compensation laws in some states are domestic workers, farmers, and employees of small companies. Workers' compensation insurance is purchased by the employer from an insurance carrier. The employer pays all premiums in return for protection from the financial liability for on-the-job injuries and illnesses.

Rehabilitation is the goal of workers' compensation insurance. Benefits provide for treatment that helps to make workers healthy enough to return to work. This includes medical and hospital care, surgery, and therapy from the time of injury or diagnosis of an illness. In the case of total or partial disability, benefits are paid to compensate for income lost. If a worker is killed on the job or dies from a job-related disease or disability, there is a moderate funeral expense allowance and living expense allowance for dependents. Benefits vary from state to state, so you should learn the workers' compensation laws in your state.

Claims for workers' compensation insurance are made with the Bureau of Workers' Compensation in each state. Since the claim forms for all states are not alike, contact the patient's employer for a copy of the proper claim form. An example of one state's workers' compensation claim form is shown in Figure 10-1.

FILING AN INSURANCE CLAIM

10.9 Assigning Payment to the Physician

Some doctors accept assignment of the patient's benefits under Medicare and other federally funded insurance programs. This means that the physician accepts the determination of the insurance carrier as

Chapter 10—Health Insurance

Figure 10-1 Workers' Compensation Claim Form

DEPARTMENT OF LABOR — WORKER'S COMPENSATION DIVISION
ATTENDING PHYSICIAN'S REPORT

The Patient
1. Name of Injured Person Andrea S. Rankin   Age 34   Sex Female
2. Address 905 Clifton Road, Atlanta, GA 30385-8893
3. Name and Address of Employer Majors Concrete Company, 238 Leaf Lane, Atlanta, GA 30342-3329

The Accident
4. Date of accident 4/9/--   Hour 3:30 p.m.   Date disability began 4/9/--
5. State in patient's own words where and how accident occurred Concrete truck backed over patient's left foot while she was pouring concrete at the construction site.

The Injury
6. Give accurate description of nature and extent of injury and state diagnosis Massive bruising to left foot; no broken bones; great deal of pain associated with bruises.
7. Will the injury result in (a) Permanent defect? No   If so, what?
   (b) Facial or head disfigurement? No
8. Is accident above referred to the only cause of patient's condition? Yes   If not, state contributing causes
9. Is patient suffering from any other disease or any disabling condition not due to this accident? No
   Give particulars
10. Has patient any physical impairment due to previous accident or disease? No   Give particulars
11. Has normal recovery been delayed for any reason? No   Give particulars

Treatment
12. Date of your first treatment 4/10/--   Who engaged your services?
13. Describe treatment given Darvon, 100 mg. q. 4h. p.r.n. for pain
14. Were X rays taken? Yes   When? 4/10/--   By Whom? Edwin Gordon, Brookville Laboratories, 2046 Lakeland Road, Atlanta, GA 30303-2993 (Name and Address)
15. X ray diagnosis No broken bones
16. Was patient treated by anyone else? No   When?   By Whom? (Name and Address)
17. Was patient hospitalized? No   Name and address of hospital
18. Date of admission to hospital   Date of discharge
19. Is further treatment needed? No   For how long?

Disability
20. Patient (was will be) able to resume (regular light) work on 4/14/--
21. If death ensued give date

REMARKS (Give any information of value not included above)

I am a duly licensed physician in the State of Georgia
I was graduated from Ohio State University   in Columbus, Ohio   Year 1956
                                                    (City, State)
Date of this report 6/21/--   (Signed) John N. Sparks, M.D.
Address 8504 Capricorn Drive, Atlanta, GA 30033-7775   Telephone 555-0078
This report must be signed personally by physician.

full payment and can collect only the amount approved by the carrier. Other doctors do not accept assignments. They ask the patient to pay for the medical expenses at the time of service and to file a claim with the insurance carrier for reimbursement. Check with your employer to learn whether assignments are accepted.

10.10 Insurance Coding Systems

CPT-4, Physicians' Current Procedural Terminology, fourth edition, lists medical procedures and treatments and provides a five-digit code to identify each procedure and treatment. Most insurance carriers recognize CPT coding as an industry standard and require use of CPT codes on claim forms. Sample procedures and treatments with their CPT codes are shown on the superbill in Figure 10-2.

ICDA — The International Classification of Diseases, Adapted is used to identify illness and disease diagnoses. Revision nine, identified as ICD-9CM, is recognized among insurance carriers as a standard for diagnosis coding. The four-digit or five-digit codes are requested on insurance claim forms to speed the processing of claims. ICDA codes are shown on the superbill in Figure 10-2.

DRGs, diagnosis-related groups, are illness groupings assigned to hospital patients. All illnesses are categorized into 467 groups, and patients are assigned to one of the groups. For example, a patient treated in the hospital for heart failure and shock is classified in DRG 157; a patient over 35 treated in the hospital for diabetes is classified in DRG 294. Originally required on Medicare claim forms, DRG codes are gaining popularity among other hospital care providers as an industry standard for coding hospital treated medical problems. Uniform payment for each hospitalized patient in a DRG is adjusted for community wage levels and is intended to cover all hospital expenses except those related to educational programs and capital improvements.

10.11 Superbill As Insurance Claim Documentation

Insurance carriers generally accept a physician's superbill as documentation for a claim. A list of procedures and treatments with their accompanying Current Procedural Terminology codes is shown on the front of the superbill. A space is provided to write the charge for each service, and additional space is provided for the physician to list the medical diagnosis. Some superbills also show ICDA codes (see Figure 10-2). When filing a superbill with an insurance claim form, complete only the top of the form (Patient/Insured Information). Figure 10-3, page 156, illustrates a superbill used with a claim form.

Chapter 10—Health Insurance **155**

Figure 10-2 Superbill with CPT and ICDA codes

DATE	DESCRIPTION	CHARGE	CREDITS		CURRENT BALANCE	PREVIOUS BALANCE	NAME	ACCT. NUMBER
			PAYMENT	ADJUSTMENT				

This is your RECEIPT for this amount ☚   ☛ This is a STATEMENT of your account to date

ATTENDING PHYSICIAN'S STATEMENT   Patient _____ Date of Service _____

DIAGNOSES ARE ICD-9-CM CODED

☐412.0	Hypertension	☐227.3	Pituitary Neoplasm		☐242.2	Hyperthyroidism
☐786.50	Chest Pain	☐193.0	Thyroid Neoplasm		☐244	Hypothyroidism
☐413.9	Angina	☐490	Bronchitis		☐240.9	Goiter
☐428.0	CHF	☐324.0	Emphysema		☐242.3	Thyroid Nodule
☐425	Cardiomyopathy	☐493.9	Asthma		☐245.9	Thyroiditis
☐427.9	Cardiac Arrhythmia	☐079.9	Viral Syndrome		☐250.9	Diabetes
		☐558.9	Gastroenteritis			

OTHER DIAGNOSIS: _____

AMA CURRENT PROCEDURAL TERMINOLOGY - 4th EDITION

1. OFFICE VISITS — New / Established — FEE
   - Limited Visit ☐90010 ☐90050
   - Intermediate Visit ☐90015 ☐90060
   - Extended Visit ☐90017 ☐90070
   - Comprehensive Visit ☐90020 ☐90080
2. HOSPITAL SERVICES
   - Hospital: ☐Metro ☐ _____
   - Admission/Hist. & Phy. ☐90220
   - Admit Date: _____ 198__
   - ICU Visits ☐90270
   - ___ visits @ ___ ea.
   - Hospital Visits ☐90260
   - ___ visits @ ___ ea.
   - Hospital Visit Limited ☐90250
   - ___ visits @ ___ ea.
   - (All Service Dates Below)
   - Date of Discharge _____ 198__
3. EMERGENCY ROOM
   - Brief Service ☐90505 ☐90540
   - Extended Service ☐90517 ☐90570
4. HOSPITAL CONSULTATIONS
   - Limited ☐90600
   - Intermediate ☐90605
   - Extended ☐90610
   - Complex ☐90620
   - Referring Physician _____
5. IMMUNIZATIONS-INJECTIONS
   - ☐TET ☐Flu ☐Pneumovax ☐90720
   - ☐Testosterone
   - ☐T-B Tine Test
   - ☐ _____

6. LABORATORY SERVICES — CPT — FEE
   - ☐Chest Xray (PA) 71010
   - ☐EKG 93000
   - ☐CBC 85021
   - ☐Urinalysis 81000
   - ☐SMAC-20 80019
   - ☐T-4 83440
   - ☐Pap Smear 88100
   - ☐Sed Rate 85650
   - ☐Occult Blood Stool 82770
   - ☐Glucose 84340
   - ☐Cholesterol 82465
   - ☐Protime 85610
   - ☐Potassium 84132
   - ☐WBC 84048
   - ☐Hemoglobin 85018
   - ☐Electrolytes 80003
   - ☐Electrolytes, BUN, CR 80005
   - ☐Thyroid Profile (T-7) 82756
   - ☐TSH 84443
   - ☐T3 RIA 84480
   - ☐Thyroid Antimicro. Antibodies 85694
   - ☐Prolactin 84146
   - ☐Testosterone 84401
   - ☐Glycohemoglobin 83020
   - ☐SMAC - 20/T4 80019
   - ☐Calcium 82310
   - ☐Triglycerides 84478
   - ☐Culture (Urine) 87086
   - ☐Sensitivity (Urine) 87086
   - ☐Culture (Throat Strep) 87060
   - ☐Lateral Skull Film 70240
   - ☐Blood Handling 99000
   - ☐24 Hour Urine For _____

7. OTHER SERVICES — FEE
   - _____
   - _____
   - _____
   - _____

TODAY'S FEES $ _____

AUTHORIZATION TO PAY PHYSICIAN DIRECT

I hereby authorize payments directly to the undersigned Physician of the Medical Benefits, if any, otherwise payable to me for his services described above. I understand that I am responsible for the charges not covered by this authorization. I hereby authorize the undersigned Physician to release any medical information necessary to process this form.

Sign _____ Date _____

PATIENTS—Insurance claims handling procedures are explained on the reverse of the Pink Copy. KEEP THIS RECORD FOR INCOME TAX AND INSURANCE CLAIM FILING.

Return: ___ Days ___ Weeks ___ Mo.
Your Next Appointment ___ / ___ / ___   AM / PM
                     Day Month Date Time

JOHN H. SPARKS, M.D.
8504 CAPRICORN DRIVE
ATLANTA, GA 30033-7775
(404) 555-0078

I.D. #20-83899022
S.S. #238-54-1345

Dates of Hospital Services
ICU Visits = ○
Hospital Visits = +
Limited = −

Mo ___ Yr ___ 1 2 3 4 5 6 7 8 9 10 11 12 13 14 15 16 17 18 19 20 21 22 23 24 25 26 27 28 29 30 31
Mo ___ Yr ___ 1 2 3 4 5 6 7 8 9 10 11 12 13 14 15 16 17 18 19 20 21 22 23 24 25 26 27 28 29 30 31

10.12 General Guidelines for Completing Claim Forms

Some physicians prefer that the medical office employee complete insurance claim forms for patients to reduce the possibility of errors. Other physicians prefer that the patient complete the top of the form and the medical office employee complete the bottom of the form when a superbill is not used as documentation.

A complete and accurate claim form can be processed routinely by insurance carriers, resulting in faster payment for the medical practice. An incomplete or inaccurate form will be rejected. Use the following guidelines as you file insurance claims. File a claim form with each

Figure 10-3 Superbill Used with Claim Form

HEALTH INSURANCE CLAIM FORM
READ INSTRUCTIONS BEFORE COMPLETING OR SIGNING THIS FORM

☐ MEDICAID ☐ MEDICARE ☐ CHAMPUS ☒ OTHER

FORM APPROVED
OMB NO. 66-R0012

PATIENT & INSURED (SUBSCRIBER) INFORMATION

1. PATIENT'S NAME (First name, middle initial, last name): John S. Hammond
2. PATIENT'S DATE OF BIRTH: 8 | 15 | --
3. INSURED'S NAME (First name, middle initial, last name): John S. Hammond
4. PATIENT'S ADDRESS (Street, city, state, ZIP code): 5168 Oak Grove Terrace, Atlanta, GA 30304-5475
5. PATIENT'S SEX: MALE ☒ FEMALE ☐
6. INSURED'S I.D. MEDICARE AND/OR MEDICAID NO. (Include any letters): 283-58-6871
7. PATIENT'S RELATIONSHIP TO INSURED: SELF ☒ SPOUSE CHILD OTHER
8. INSURED'S GROUP NO. (Or Group Name): TN 75281
TELEPHONE NO.
9. OTHER HEALTH INSURANCE COVERAGE — Enter Name of Policyholder and Plan Name and Address and Policy or Medical Assistance Number: None
10. WAS CONDITION RELATED TO:
   A. PATIENT'S EMPLOYMENT: YES ☐ NO ☒
   B. ACCIDENT: AUTO ☐ OTHER ☐
11. INSURED'S ADDRESS (Street, city, state, ZIP code): 5168 Oak Grove Terrace, Atlanta, GA 30304-5475
12. PATIENT'S OR AUTHORIZED PERSON'S SIGNATURE (Read back before signing) I Authorize the Release of any Medical Information Necessary to Process this Claim and Request Payment of MEDICARE Benefits Either to Myself or to the Party Who Accepts Assignment Below
SIGNED _____ DATE _____
13. I AUTHORIZE PAYMENT OF MEDICAL BENEFITS TO UNDERSIGNED PHYSICIAN OR SUPPLIER FOR SERVICE DESCRIBED BELOW
SIGNED (Insured or Authorized Person) _____

PHYSICIAN OR SUPPLIER INFORMATION

14. DATE OF: ILLNESS (FIRST SYMPTOM) OR INJURY (ACCIDENT) OR PREGNANCY (LMP)
15. DATE FIRST CONSULTED YOU FOR THIS CONDITION
16. HAS PATIENT EVER HAD SAME OR SIMILAR SYMPTOMS? YES ☐ NO ☒
16a. IF AN EMERGENCY CHECK HERE ☐

DATE	DESCRIPTION	CHARGE	CREDITS PAYMENT	ADJUSTMENT	CURRENT BALANCE	PREVIOUS BALANCE	NAME	ACCT. NUMBER
4/14/--	O.V., Lab, Xray	100.00			100.00	---	John S. Hammond	839

This is your RECEIPT for this amount
This is a STATEMENT of your account to date

ATTENDING PHYSICIAN'S STATEMENT   Patient _John Hammond_   Date of Service _4/14/--_

DIAGNOSES ARE ICD-9-CM CODED

☒ 412.0	Hypertension	☐ 227.3	Pituitary Neoplasm	☐ 242.2	Hyperthyroidism
☒ 786.50	Chest Pain	☐ 193.0	Thyroid Neoplasm	☐ 244	Hypothyroidism
☒ 413.9	Angina	☐ 490	Bronchitis	☐ 240.9	Goiter
☐ 428.0	CHF	☐ 324.0	Emphysema	☐ 242.3	Thyroid Nodule
☐ 425	Cardiomyopathy	☐ 493.9	Asthma	☐ 245.9	Thyroiditis
☐ 427.9	Cardiac Arrhythmia	☐ 079.9	Viral Syndrome	☐ 250.9	Diabetes
		☐ 558.9	Gastroenteritis		

OTHER DIAGNOSIS: _Hypoglycemia (251.0)_

AMA CURRENT PROCEDURAL TERMINOLOGY - 4th EDITION

1. OFFICE VISITS — New / Established / FEE
   Limited Visit ☐ 90010 ☐ 90050
   Intermediate Visit ☐ 90015 ☒ 90060 25.00
   Extended Visit ☐ 90017 ☐ 90070
   Comprehensive Visit ☐ 90020 ☐ 90080

2. HOSPITAL SERVICES
   Hospital: ☐ Metro ☐
   Admission/Hist. & Phy. ☐ 90220
   Admit Date: ____ 198__
   ICU Visits ☐ 90270
   ____ visits @ ____ ea.
   Hospital Visits ☐ 90260
   ____ visits @ ____ ea.
   Hospital Visit Limited ☐ 90250
   ____ visits @ ____ ea.
   (All Service Dates Below)
   Date of Discharge ____ 198__

3. EMERGENCY ROOM
   Brief Service ☐ 90505 ☐ 90540
   Extended Service ☐ 90517 ☐ 90570

4. HOSPITAL CONSULTATIONS
   Limited ☐ 90600
   Intermediate ☐ 90605
   Extended ☐ 90610
   Complex ☐ 90620
   Referring Physician ____

5. IMMUNIZATIONS-INJECTIONS
   ☐ TET ☐ Flu ☐ Pneumovax ☐ 90720
   ☐ Testosterone
   ☐ T-B Tine Test

6. LABORATORY SERVICES — CPT — FEE
   ☒ Chest Xray (PA) 71010 30.00
   ☒ EKG 93000 30.00
   ☐ CBC 85021
   ☐ Urinalysis 81000
   ☐ SMAC-20 80019
   ☐ T-4 83440
   ☐ Pap Smear 88100
   ☐ Sed Rate 85650
   ☐ Occult Blood Stool 82770
   ☐ Glucose 84340
   ☐ Cholesterol 82465
   ☐ Protime 85610
   ☐ Potassium 84132
   ☐ WBC 84048
   ☐ Hemoglobin 85018
   ☒ Electrolytes 80003 15.00
   ☐ Electrolytes, BUN, CR 80005
   ☐ Thyroid Profile (T-7) 82756
   ☐ TSH 84443
   ☐ T3 RIA 84480
   ☐ Thyroid Antimicro. Antibodies 85694
   ☐ Prolactin 84146
   ☐ Testosterone 84401
   ☐ Glycohemoglobin 83020
   ☐ SMAC - 20/T4 80019
   ☐ Calcium 82310
   ☐ Triglycerides 84478
   ☐ Culture (Urine) 87086
   ☐ Sensitivity (Urine) 87086
   ☐ Culture (Throat Strep) 87060
   ☐ Lateral Skull Film 70240
   ☐ Blood Handling 99000

7. OTHER SERVICES — FEE
   ____

TODAY'S FEES $ 100.00

AUTHORIZATION TO PAY PHYSICIAN DIRECT
I hereby authorize payments directly to the undersigned Physician of the Medical Benefits, if any, otherwise payable to me for his services described above. I understand that I am responsible for the charges not covered by this authorization. I hereby authorize the undersigned Physician to release any medical information necessary to process this form.
Sign _____ Date _____
PATIENTS—Insurance claims handling procedures are explained on the reverse of the Pink Copy. KEEP THIS RECORD FOR INCOME TAX AND INSURANCE CLAIM FILING.

Return: ____ Days ____ Weeks ____ Mo.
Your Next Appointment ____ / ____ / ____ AM/PM
                        Day   Month   Date   Time

JOHN H. SPARKS, M.D.

insurance carrier providing coverage for the patient. Though the forms required by the various carriers differ in some ways, the guidelines are important when filing a claim with any carrier.

1. Complete each line of the claim form. Write legibly or type the form.
2. Type *DNA* (does not apply) on any lines which do not apply to the claim.
3. Provide complete information about procedures, treatments, and diagnoses.
4. Give procedure and treatment codes and diagnosis codes.
5. List DRG for hospital patients.
6. List all dates accurately.
7. Obtain all necessary signatures.
8. Check for agreement of diagnoses and treatments.
9. List all charges. Do not summarize.
10. Provide accurate totals.
11. Double check the insurance policy number.
12. Submit forms to the proper administering agency.
13. Submit forms to all carriers which provide coverage to the patient.
14. Provide a detailed report of nonstandard treatments.
15. List each service separately for each visit.
16. Group office and hospital visits together if the fee is the same for each visit.
17. Itemize laboratory work separately from office visits.
18. Itemize injections separately.
19. Itemize X rays separately.
20. Provide detailed information regarding excision of tumors. List the type, number, category, size, weight, and location of tumors.
21. Provide detailed information regarding lacerations. List the length, location, and type of repair.
22. Itemize special materials.
23. List federal identification numbers and provider identification numbers.
24. Submit claims to the insurance carrier promptly.
25. File a copy of the claim form in the patient's medical record.
26. Establish an audit trail for the claim (see Section 10.14).

10.13 AMA Universal Health Insurance Claim Form

A Universal Health Insurance Claim Form, developed by the American Medical Association, has been adopted for use by most group and individual health insurance claim organizations and by many of the administrators of government health insurance programs, including Medicare, Medicaid, and CHAMPUS/CHAMPVA. Even though some of these organizations include their name and logo on the form, giving it the appearance of a special form, the universal form is shown in the body of the document.

The Universal Health Insurance Claim Form is divided into two major sections: patient information and physician information. The patient/subscriber section contains 11 spaces for information and 2 spaces for signatures. The physician/supplier section consists of 20 spaces for information, but they are not all used for each claim. A space is given for the physician's signature.

A description of each space and its relevance to Medicare, Medicaid, and private insurance carriers is given below. For Blue Shield claims, refer to the local plan. A completed Universal Health Insurance Claim Form is shown in Figure 10-4.

The numbered items below correspond to the numbered spaces on the claim form.

1. Type the patient's name.

2. Type the patient's birth date in numerals; for example, September 15, 1941, should be typed 9/15/41. For Medicare, type *DNA*.

3. Type the insured's name (the name of the person to whom the policy was issued). If the insured and the patient are the same, you may type *same*. For Medicare, type *DNA*.

4. Type the patient's full address. Place the street address on the first line and the city, state, and ZIP code on the second line.

5. Mark the correct box to indicate the patient's sex.

6. Type the patient's insurance identification number, Medicare number, or Medicaid number, including any letters which are part of the identification. Include numbers from all applicable insurance programs. Ask the patient for an insurance identification card which shows the complete number. For Medicare, use the number on the beneficiary's red, white, and blue health insurance card. The Medicaid I.D. number is assigned by the local agency. For Blue Shield, use the number on the subscriber's identification card which is usually referred to as the "Identification" or "Certification" or "Contract" number.

7. Mark the correct box indicating the patient's relationship to the insured.

Chapter 10—Health Insurance 159

Figure 10-4 Universal Health Insurance Claim Form

HEALTH INSURANCE CLAIM FORM
READ INSTRUCTIONS BEFORE COMPLETING OR SIGNING THIS FORM

☐ MEDICAID ☐ MEDICARE ☐ CHAMPUS ☒ OTHER

FORM APPROVED
OMB NO. 66-R0012

PATIENT & INSURED (SUBSCRIBER) INFORMATION

1. PATIENT'S NAME (First name, middle initial, last name)
John S. Hammond

2. PATIENT'S DATE OF BIRTH
08 | 15 | 41

3. INSURED'S NAME (First name, middle initial, last name)
John S. Hammond

4. PATIENT'S ADDRESS (Street, city, state, ZIP code)
5168 Oak Grove Terrace
Decatur, Georgia 30033-8823
TELEPHONE NO

5. PATIENT'S SEX
MALE ☒ FEMALE ☐

6. INSURED'S I.D. MEDICARE AND/OR MEDICAID NO (Include any letters)
283-58-6871

7. PATIENT'S RELATIONSHIP TO INSURED
SELF ☒ SPOUSE ☐ CHILD ☐ OTHER ☐

8. INSURED'S GROUP NO (Or Group Name)
TN 75281

9. OTHER HEALTH INSURANCE COVERAGE - Enter Name of Policyholder and Plan Name and Address and Policy or Medical Assistance Number
John Hammond; United Surgical Plan; 53 Taft Road, Nashville, TN 37206-1293; Group No. 6248

10. WAS CONDITION RELATED TO
A. PATIENT'S EMPLOYMENT
YES ☐ NO ☒
B. ACCIDENT
AUTO ☐ OTHER ☒

11. INSURED'S ADDRESS (Street, city, state, ZIP code)
5168 Oak Grove Terrace
Decatur, GA 30033-8823

12. PATIENT'S OR AUTHORIZED PERSON'S SIGNATURE (Read back before signing)
I Authorize the Release of any Medical Information Necessary to Process this Claim and Request Payment of MEDICARE Benefits Either to Myself or to the Party Who Accepts Assignment Below
SIGNED *John S. Hammond* DATE 6/16/--

13. I AUTHORIZE PAYMENT OF MEDICAL BENEFITS TO UNDERSIGNED PHYSICIAN OR SUPPLIER FOR SERVICE DESCRIBED BELOW
SIGNED *John S. Hammond* (Insured or Authorized Person)

PHYSICIAN OR SUPPLIER INFORMATION

14. DATE OF
2/25/--

15. ILLNESS (FIRST SYMPTOM) OR INJURY (ACCIDENT) OR PREGNANCY (LMP)

15. DATE FIRST CONSULTED YOU FOR THIS CONDITION
4/14/--

16. HAS PATIENT EVER HAD SAME OR SIMILAR SYMPTOMS?
YES ☒ NO ☐

16a. IF AN EMERGENCY CHECK HERE ☐ DNA

17. DATE PATIENT ABLE TO RETURN TO WORK
DNA

18. DATES OF TOTAL DISABILITY
FROM DNA THROUGH DNA

DATES OF PARTIAL DISABILITY
FROM DNA THROUGH DNA

19. NAME OF REFERRING PHYSICIAN OR OTHER SOURCE (e.g. public health agency)
Ann Kirkpatrick, M.D.

20. FOR SERVICES RELATED TO HOSPITALIZATION GIVE HOSPITALIZATION DATES
ADMITTED DNA DISCHARGED DNA

21. NAME & ADDRESS OF FACILITY WHERE SERVICES RENDERED (If other than home or office)
DNA

22. WAS LABORATORY WORK PERFORMED OUTSIDE YOUR OFFICE?
YES ☒ NO ☐ CHARGES DNA

23. DIAGNOSIS OR NATURE OF ILLNESS OR INJURY. RELATE DIAGNOSIS TO PROCEDURE IN COLUMN D BY REFERENCE NUMBERS 1, 2, 3 ETC OR DX CODE
1. Unstable arteriosclerotic heart disease, recent
2. heart irregularity (412.9)
3. Type II hypoglycemia (251.0)

B. EPSDT FAMILY PLANNING
YES ☐ DNA NO ☐
YES ☐ DNA NO ☐

PRIOR AUTHORIZATION NO _____

24.A DATE OF SERVICE	B PLACE OF SERVICE	C PROCEDURE CODE (IDENTIFY)	FULLY DESCRIBE PROCEDURES, MEDICAL SERVICES OR SUPPLIES FURNISHED FOR EACH DATE GIVEN (EXPLAIN UNUSUAL SERVICES OR CIRCUMSTANCES)	D DIAGNOSIS CODE	E CHARGES	F DAYS OR UNITS	G TOS	H LEAVE BLANK
4/14/--	3	90060	Intermediate service	412.9 251.0	25 00			
4/14/--	3	71020	Chest X ray	412.9	30 00			
4/14/--	3	93000	Electrocardiogram	412.9	30 00			
4/14/--	3	80003	Blood sugar check	251.0	15 00			

25. SIGNATURE OF PHYSICIAN OR SUPPLIER
(I certify that the statements on the reverse apply to this bill and are made a part hereof)
SIGNED *John H. Sparks, M.D.* DATE 6/16/--

26. ACCEPT ASSIGNMENT (GOVERNMENT CLAIMS ONLY) (SEE BACK)
YES ☒ NO ☐

27. TOTAL CHARGE
100.00

28. AMOUNT PAID
None

29. BALANCE DUE
$100 00

30. YOUR SOCIAL SECURITY NO
238-54-1345

31. PHYSICIAN'S OR SUPPLIER'S NAME, ADDRESS, ZIP CODE & TELEPHONE NO
John H. Sparks, M.D.
8504 Capricorn Drive
Atlanta, GA 30033-7775
(404) 555-0078

32. YOUR PATIENT'S ACCOUNT
839

33. YOUR EMPLOYER I.D. NO
2083899022

PLACE OF SERVICE AND TYPE OF SERVICE (T O S) CODES ON THE BACK
REMARKS

APPROVED BY AMA COUNCIL ON MEDICAL SERVICE 5-80
APPROVED BY THE HEALTH CARE FINANCING ADMINISTRATION & CHAMPUS

Form **AMA-OP-407**
Form **HCFA-1500 (4-80)**
Form **CHAMPUS-501**

8. Type the identification number of the insured's group, if this is a group claim, or the name of the patient's health maintenance organization. If patient is not covered by group insurance, type *DNA*.

9. If the file indicates the patient is covered by any other health insurance, type the name of the policyholder, the name of the insurance company, the address of the insurance company, and the policy number. This includes but is not limited to Medicare, Medicaid, Federal Health Insurance Benefits, CHAMPUS or CHAMPVA. If the file shows no record of any other health insurance coverage, type *DNA*.

10. **A.,B.** Mark the proper boxes indicating the cause of the patient's condition. For Medicare, type *DNA* for 10B.

11. Type the insured's full address. For Medicare, type *DNA*.

12,
13. Secure the patient's signature or the signature of the patient's parent or guardian. The signature in box 12 gives the patient's permission for the physician to release medical information to the insurance carrier. A signature in box 13 gives the patient's permission for the insurance company to pay the physician directly. When an illiterate or physically handicapped enrollee signs by marking an x, a witness should sign next to the mark and enter an address.

14. Type the date of the first symptoms of an illness or the date of an injury. If the reason for the visit was a suspected pregnancy, write the date of the last menstrual period (LMP).

15. Type the date of the patient's first visit to the physician for the condition named on the claim form. For Medicare, type *DNA*.

16. Mark the appropriate box. Type the dates of previous symptoms on a separate sheet and attach. If this was an emergency visit, check 16A. For Medicare, type *DNA*.

17. If the patient will receive disability benefits, complete this box; otherwise, type *DNA*. For Medicare, type *DNA*.

18. Complete this blank if the patient will receive disability benefits; otherwise, type *DNA*. For Medicare, type *DNA*.

19. Type the referring physician's name for first consultation; thereafter, type *DNA*. If there is no referring physician, type *DNA*. For Medicare, complete for each claim involving a referral.

20. Complete this box if patient was hospitalized; otherwise, type *DNA*.

21. If services were rendered outside the physician's office or the patient's home, type the name and address of the person or facility providing the service. If not, type *DNA*.

22. Answer the question. If laboratory work was done, type the charges. If there are no charges, type *DNA*.

23. A. Look at the medical record or the superbill to determine the diagnosis(es). Type the diagnosis and diagnosis codes. Identify the code used, commonly ICD-9CM, in the heading of 24D.

   B. For Medicare, leave this blank. For Medicaid, the blocks for *EPSDT* (Early and Periodic Screening for Diagnosis and Treatment of Children) and *Family Planning* are used to indicate whether these services are involved. If so, funds especially designated for these purposes will be used for reimbursement. *Prior authorization* is required for certain services that Medicaid will not reimburse without prior approval. A special number is issued for prior authorizations, and it must be entered on the form before payment will be made for the services in question.

24. To complete Section 24, type across the page. Complete each column of Line 1 before going to Line 2.

   A. List the date of service shown in the medical record or on the superbill. If *From* and *To* are used for a series of identical services, the number of these services should be shown in Column *F*. Continue to Column *B*.

   B. From the *place of service* codes shown at the bottom or on the back of the form, type the number or letters corrresponding to the place where the service was performed. Continue to Column *C*. For Blue Shield, type the number to indicate place of service. For Medicare, only the Alpha Codes shown in parentheses on the back of the form should be used. If the physician is billing for a lab service performed in the office, code *O* (Doctor's Office) should be used. If the physician is billing for a lab service purchased from another physician who maintains a lab, code *OL* (Other Location) should be shown. If the physician is billing for a lab service purchased from an independent lab, code *IL* should be used. Spaces 21 and 22 must be completed for all laboratory work performed outside of the physician's office. Claims for ambulance service (Code 9) for Medicare beneficiaries should be made on form SSA-1491. Alpha Codes *RTC* and *STF* are not used for Medicare.

   C. The information for this section is given on the superbill and in the medical record. Identify the procedure code being used, commonly CPT-4, by typing the name of the code in the heading of 24C. Type the code for the first procedure. This is likely to be a routine office visit called *intermediate service*. The CPT-4 code for intermediate service for an established patient is 90060. Explain any unusual circumstances to help process the claim.

In the next column of this section, type the description of the procedure. In the example, "Intermediate Service" matches the procedure code 90060.

- D. Refer to Section 23 of the claim form. Use the numbers 1, 2, 3, 4, or the diagnosis codes shown in Section 23 to relate the date of service and the procedures to the appropriate diagnosis.
- E. From the physician's fee schedule, determine the fee for each procedure. Type the amount in the *Charges* column. Proceed to line 2 of box 24. Continue across the page and complete each column as you did for line 1.
- F. For Medicare: If *From* and *To* dates are entered in Column *A* for a series of identical services, give the number of services here.
- G. For Medicare: List the type of service code listed on the back of the form. These may be adjusted by the Medicare carrier.
- H. For Medicare and Blue Shield: The blank space has been provided for Medicare and Blue Shield. Refer to your local administrator.
  For Medicare: If the physician provides a superbill, it may be used instead of Section 24.

25. The physician or a person designated by the physician must sign and date the form.
26. Mark the correct box to indicate whether the physician accepts assignments of benefits under government-funded programs. This does not include the Federal Employee Program and does not refer to Medicaid.
27. Type the amount of the total charge.
28. Type any amount which was paid by another source, such as another carrier. If none was paid by another source, type *none*.
29. Type the balance due.
30. Type the physician's Social Security number.
31. Type the physician's full address and telephone number. This information may be preprinted or rubber stamped. The *I.D. No.* should be used when the physician or supplier is employed by a health maintenance organization which has assigned the physician a special number or when the physician is identified by a special number for administrators of other programs.
32. Type the patient's account number. If none, type *DNA*.
33. Type the physician's identification number (if there is one) when the physician or supplier is providing services in a group practice or is employed by a hospital or other institution which has assigned an *Employer I.D. No.*

Copy the form for the medical office files. Send the original to the insurance carrier.

10.14 Audit Trails

An *audit trail* should be established to follow up all insurance claims. Since much of the income from a medical practice comes from insurance carriers, proper follow-up is necessary to maintain the stability of financial operations. Use one of the two methods described below for effective follow-up of claims.

Claim Register. Use a *claim register* to record important information about each claim. Show the name of each patient for which a claim is submitted, the date the claim is submitted to the carrier, and the amount of the claim. Show the date the claim is paid and the amount paid. Indicate any difference between the two. Give a follow-up date for six weeks in the future. If the claim is unpaid after six weeks, begin the follow-up procedure described below. A claim register is shown in Figure 10-5.

Figure 10-5 Claim Register

INSURANCE CLAIMS REGISTER

	Claim No.	Patient	Carrier	Claim Submitted Date	Claim Submitted Amount	Follow-up Date	Claim Paid Date	Claim Paid Amount	Difference (Submitted - Paid)	
1	601	Clara Vinings	Liberty Mutual	5/17	62.00	6/30	6/2	54.00	8.00	1
2	602	Jason Martin	Blue Shield	5/17	26.00	6/30	6/15	20.00	6.00	2
3	603	Anthony Garcia	Nationwide	5/18	78.00	6/30				3
4	604	Barbara Cosby	Aetna Life + Casualty	5/18	26.00	6/30	6/4	26.00	—	4
5	605	Gerard Jackson	Blue Shield	5/23	84.00	7/7				5
6										6
7										7
8										8
9										9
10										10
11										11
12										12
13										13
14										14
15										15

Tickler File. Maintain a *tickler file* of pending claims. As you submit an insurance claim, file a copy of the claim in a folder dated six weeks into the future. (If you submit a claim on June 1, file the copy of the claim form in the folder for July 15.) When a claim is paid, record the payment on the patient's ledger card; then remove the copy of the claim form from the tickler file. (Another copy should already be filed in the patient's medical record.) At the end of the billing period, review all the claim forms in the tickler file to determine which claims are due but remain unpaid. Begin the follow-up procedure described below. A tickler file is shown in Figure 10-6.

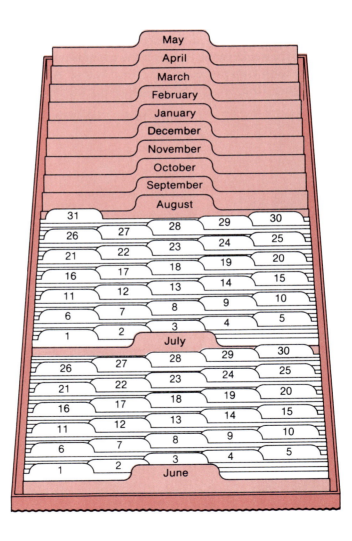

Figure 10-6 Tickler File

Follow-up Procedure. If payment has not been received, write a follow-up letter to the insurance company asking for payment and enclose a copy of the claim form. If you are using a claim register, enter the date of this letter and note a follow-up date six weeks in the future. If you are using a tickler file, attach a copy of this letter to the file copy of the claim form and return it to the tickler file, once again in a folder dated six weeks in the future. Continue with this collections process until the claim is paid.

REFERENCES

American Medical Association, Division of Medical Practice. AMA Health Insurance Claim Form, revised 1980.

CHAMPUS Instructions for Use of the AMA Health Insurance Claim Form. Chicago: American Medical Association.

Physicians' Current Procedural Terminology, 4th ed. Chicago: American Medical Association, 1984.

K. F. Gow and B. R. Ricks. *Medical and Dental Associates, P.C.* Cincinnati: South-Western Publishing Co., 1985.

11

Accounting Procedures in the Medical Office

PEGBOARD ACCOUNTING

A simple write-it-once method of handling financial transactions in a medical office is called *pegboard accounting,* named for the pegboard on which the accounting papers are prepared. By using pegboard accounting, charges and credits can be posted on several different records in one operation. By posting all the entries at once, the probability of making errors is reduced.

The three elements of a pegboard accounting system are (1) the superbill, (2) the patient ledger card, and (3) the daily financial log. Commercially prepared pegboard accounting materials composed of these three elements are available from medical office supply companies.

11.1 Superbill

The *superbill,* or patient charge slip, is a comprehensive listing of examinations, procedures, and treatments which a patient might receive from a medical office, plus the fee for each of these services. Superbills are numbered sequentially, similar to the numbering of checks in a checkbook. When a patient registers at the reception desk, the receptionist assembles the next numbered superbill, the ledger card, and the daily log (See Section 11.4). The receptionist then writes the date, the previous balance, the patient's name, and the patient's number, if used, on the superbill. In a pegboard accounting system, the information recorded on the superbill is automatically posted to the ledger card and the daily log. The superbill is clipped to the medical record and follows the patient from the time of registration until after the examination is completed.

During the examination, the physician marks the superbill to indicate the procedure or treatment performed and to say how soon the

Chapter 11—Accounting Procedures in the Medical Office   **167**

patient should return. The doctor gives the superbill to the patient or nurse when the examination is complete, and the patient or nurse returns it to the receptionist. Based on the established fees for the procedure or treatment, the receptionist computes patient charges and records them in the proper columns of the superbill. Any payments or adjustments are also recorded. By referring to the highlighted information in Figure 11-1, you will see that Romero Sanchez had a previous balance of $25 at the beginning of his visit to the doctor. To this amount was added $25 for an office visit and $15 for lab work. Mr. Sanchez made a payment of $30 and has an outstanding balance of $35. As these amounts are recorded on the superbill, they are automatically transferred to the ledger card and daily log.

Figure 11-1   Superbill

DATE	DESCRIPTION	CHARGE	CREDITS		CURRENT BALANCE	PREVIOUS BALANCE	NAME	ACCT. NUMBER
			PAYMENT	ADJUSTMENT				
6/14/--	O.V., Lab	40.00	30.00		35.00	25.00	Romero Sanchez	407

This is your RECEIPT for this amount
ATTENDING PHYSICIAN'S STATEMENT
This is a STATEMENT of your account to date
Patient _Romero Sanchez_   Date of Service _6/14/--_

DIAGNOSES ARE ICD-9-CM CODED

☐ 412.0	Hypertension	☐ 227.3	Pituitary Neoplasm		☐ 242.2	Hyperthyroidism	
☐ 786.50	Chest Pain	☐ 193.0	Thyroid Neoplasm		☐ 244	Hypothyroidism	
☐ 413.9	Angina	☐ 490	Bronchitis		☐ 240.9	Goiter	
☐ 428.0	C H F	☐ 324.0	Emphysema		☐ 242.3	Thyroid Nodule	
☐ 425	Cardiomyopathy	☐ 493.9	Asthma		☐ 245.9	Thyroiditis	
☐ 427.9	Cardiac Arrhythmia	☐ 079.9	Viral Syndrome		☐ 250.9	Diabetes	
		☐ 558.9	Gastroenteritis				

OTHER DIAGNOSIS: _Anemia_

AMA CURRENT PROCEDURAL TERMINOLOGY - 4th EDITION

1. OFFICE VISITS	New	Established	FEE	6. LABORATORY SERVICES	CPT	FEE	7. OTHER SERVICES	FEE
Limited Visit	☐ 90010	☐ 90050		☐ Chest Xray (PA)	71010			
Intermediate Visit	☐ 90015	☑ 90060	25.00	☐ EKG	93000			
Extended Visit	☐ 90017	☐ 90070		☑ CBC	85021	15.00		
Comprehensive Visit	☐ 90020	☐ 90080		☐ Urinalysis	81000			
2. HOSPITAL SERVICES				☐ SMAC-20	80019			
Hospital: ☐ Metro ☐				☐ T-4	83440			
Admission/Hist. & Phy. ☐ 90220				☐ Pap Smear	88100			
Admit Date: ____198__				☐ Sed Rate	85650		TODAY'S FEES	$ 40.00
ICU Visits ☐ 90270				☐ Occult Blood Stool	82770			
____visits @ ____ ea.				☐ Glucose	84340			
Hospital Visits ☐ 90260				☐ Cholesterol	82465		AUTHORIZATION TO PAY PHYSICIAN DIRECT	
____visits @ ____ ea.				☐ Protime	85610			
Hospital Visits Limited ☐ 90250				☐ Potassium	84132		I hereby authorize payments directly to the undersigned Physician of the Medical Benefits, if any, otherwise payable to me for his services described above. I understand that I am responsible for the charges not covered by this authorization. I hereby authorize the undersigned Physician to release any medical information necessary to process this form.	
____visits @ ____ ea.				☐ WBC	84048			
(All Service Dates Below)				☐ Hemoglobin	85018			
Date of Discharge ____ 198__				☐ Electrolytes	80003			
3. EMERGENCY ROOM				☐ Electrolytes, BUN, CR	80005			
Brief Service	☐ 90505	☐ 90540		☐ Thyroid Profile (T-7)	82756			
Extended Service	☐ 90517	☐ 90570		☐ TSH	84443		Sign ____ Date ____	
				☐ T3 RIA	84480		PATIENTS—Insurance claims handling procedures are explained on the reverse of the Pink Copy KEEP THIS RECORD FOR INCOME TAX AND INSURANCE CLAIM FILING	
4. HOSPITAL CONSULTATIONS				☐ Thyroid Antimicro Antibodies	85694			
Limited		☐ 90600		☐ Prolactin	84146			
Intermediate		☐ 90605		☐ Testosterone	84401			
Extended		☐ 90610		☐ Glycohemoglobin	83020			
Complex		☐ 90620		☐ SMAC - 20/T4	80019		Return ___ Days ___ Weeks ___ Mo	
Referring Physician ____				☐ Calcium	82310		Your Next Appointment ____	AM PM
				☐ Triglycerides	84478		Day Month Date Time	
5. IMMUNIZATIONS-INJECTIONS				☐ Culture (Urine)	87086			
☐ TET ☐ Flu ☐ Pneumavax		☐ 90720		☐ Sensitivity (Urine)	87086			
☐ Testosterone				☐ Culture (Throat Strep)	87060			
☐ T-B Tine Test				☐ Lateral Skull Film	70240			
☐				☐ Blood Handling	99000		**JOHN H. SPARKS, M.D.**	
				☐ 24 Hour Urine For ____			8504 CAPRICORN DRIVE ATLANTA, GA 30033-7775 (404) 555-0078	
Dates of Hospital Services	Mo Yr	1 2 3 4 5 6 7 8 9 10 11 12 13 14 15 16 17 18 19 20 21 22 23 24 25 26 27 28 29 30 31						
ICU Visits = O Hospital Visits = + Limited = -	Mo Yr	1 2 3 4 5 6 7 8 9 10 11 12 13 14 15 16 17 18 19 20 21 22 23 24 25 26 27 28 29 30 31					I.D. #20-83899022 S.S. #238-54-1345	

Current Procedural Terminology, Fourth Edition (CPT-4), codes are used by most insurance companies as the standard identification for medical procedures (see Section 10.10). When the five-digit CPT-4 codes and the name of the accompanying procedures are printed on a superbill, they can be marked to indicate the procedures performed for each patient. The properly marked superbill is accepted by most insurance companies as documentation for a claim.

The codes and procedures printed on superbills differ from specialty to specialty because the procedures used in each specialty are different. The most common procedures performed in the specialty area are listed. Figure 11-1 illustrates a superbill from a practice of internal medicine.

11.2 Ledger Card

The *ledger card* lists chronologically all financial activity involving one patient's account over a period of time. The ledger card is placed beneath a superbill on the pegboard; then, as the superbill is completed, the information is automatically transferred to the ledger card. Information recorded on a ledger card includes the following: (1) the dates of the doctor's services, (2) the charge for each of the procedures performed, (3) all payments by check, (4) all payments by cash, (5) any adjustments made to the bill (such as an overcharge or an overpayment), and (6) the balance remaining after payments are subtracted from charges.

Payments made by mail and charges for hospital visits are also recorded on the ledger card. A single ledger card is used for recording all financial transactions until the card is full; then a new card is begun for the patient. In Figure 11-2, the highlighted information illustrates the information which was automatically transferred to the ledger card from the superbill.

11.3 Daily Log

The *daily log* is a complete record of each day's financial activity. As charges and payments for each patient are recorded on the superbill and ledger card, they are automatically posted to the daily log as well. Charges for hospital visits and payments by mail are also transferred to the daily log when they are recorded on the ledger card, even though the patient is not seen at the office. A separate log is kept for each day. At the end of the day, each column on the daily log is totaled in order to summarize the day's financial activity. Other financial information can be included on the log, such as week-to-date or month-to-date summaries, daily bank deposit information, or summaries of each phy-

Chapter 11—Accounting Procedures in the Medical Office

Figure 11-2 Ledger Card

LEDGER SHEET
JOHN H. SPARKS, M.D.

Romero Sanchez 407
253-A Lost Creek Circle
Atlanta, GA 30033-2289

DATE	DESCRIPTION	CHARGE	CREDITS		CURRENT BALANCE
			PAYMENT	ADJUSTMENT	
4/17/--	O.V., Xray	55.00	30.00		25.00
6/14/--	O.V., Lab	40.00	30.00		35.00

sician's daily financial activity. In Figure 11-3, the highlighted information illustrates the information which was automatically transferred to the daily log from Romero Sanchez's superbill and ledger card.

Figure 11-3 Daily Log

INTERNAL MEDICINE			DAILY LOG					(404) 555-00"
			John H. Sparks, M.D. 8504 Capricorn Drive Atlanta, GA 30033-7775					
DATE	DESCRIPTION	CHARGE	CREDITS PAYMENT	ADJUSTMENT	CURRENT BALANCE	PREVIOUS BALANCE	NAME	ACCT NUMB
6/14/--	O.V., EKG, LAB	70.00			70.00	——	Susan Hall	490
6/14/--	O.V., Xray	55.00	55.00		0.00	——	Lori Learner	629
6/14/--	Hosp. Visit	60.00			320.00	260.00	Arthur Cook	505
6/14/--	O.V., EKG	55.00	25.00		30.00	——	Norris Littrell	870
6/14/--	O.V., LAB	59.00	15.00		124.00	80.00	Samuel King	741
6/14/--	O.V., EKG	55.00	55.00		0.00	——	James Scott	799
6/14/--	Hosp. Visit	75.00			265.00	190.00	Rudolf Gold	540
6/14/--	O.V., LAB	40.00	15.00		25.00	——	Jessica Rome	682
6/14/--	O.V., LAB	40.00	30.00		35.00	25.00	Romero Sanchez	407
TOTALS								

11.4 Guidelines for Completing Financial Records

By using the three pegboard accounting elements described in Sections 11.1-11.3, it is possible to complete a patient financial transaction in one writing. Complete the following steps to record transactions.

Beginning Activities. Refer to Figure 11-4 as you review beginning pegboard accounting activities.

1. At the beginning of each day, attach a new daily log to the accounting pegboard.
2. Place the writing line of the first patient's superbill over the first blank line of the daily log. Make certain the headings on the superbill are aligned correctly with the same headings on the daily log. The carbonized back of the superbill or a special carbonless paper allows print to transfer from the superbill to the daily log.
3. Write (1) the day's date, (2) the name of the patient, (3) the patient's number, if used, and (4) the patient's previous balance (from the patient's ledger card). If there is no previous balance, draw a line in the Previous Balance column.
4. Attach the superbill to the front of the patient's medical record and put the medical record in a set location where the nurse can find it. The nurse will deliver the medical record and the superbill to the physician.
5. When the next patient arrives, place the writing line of a new superbill on the next blank line of the daily log and follow Steps 3 and 4. Continue using superbills in this manner for all patients.

Figure 11-4 shows a daily log with an attached superbill. Notice that the superbill is placed directly beneath the last entry line.

Ending Activities. After the patient or nurse returns to the receptionist with the superbill, complete these steps. Refer to Figure 11-5 as you complete the superbill.

1. Place the patient's ledger card in the correct position on the daily log. Align the first blank line of the ledger card with the patient's name, which was transferred to the daily log from the superbill when the person registered. Align the columns of the ledger card with the columns of the daily log.
2. Place the superbill over the ledger card. Align the columns of the superbill with the columns of the ledger card.
3. Note the procedures indicated on the superbill by the physician or nurse. Write the fees your practice charges for these procedures beside the name of the procedure. Add all the fees to obtain a total charge.

Figure 11-4 Daily Log and Superbill

Figure 11-5 Superbill, Ledger Card, and Daily Log Completed for Ending Activities

4. Write the fee totals in the *Charges* column of the superbill.

5. In the *Credits* section of the form, write the amount that the patient has paid, plus any adjustments (for previous overcharges).

6. Find the *Current Balance* by following the steps listed below:

   a. Subtract today's credits from today's charges.

   b. Add the remainder (if there is one) to the previous balance.

   c. Write the Current Balance in the correct column. If the Current Balance is zero, draw a line through the *Current Balance* column.

7. Give the superbill to the patient. The superbill serves as a statement and as documentation for an insurance claim.

8. File the ledger card in the ledger card file.

11.5 Recording Charges for Hospital Visits

The following three methods are generally used for recording charges for hospital visits: (1) In some medical offices, hospital visits are recorded daily on the patient's ledger card and on the daily log; no daily superbill is used. At the time of the patient's discharge, a superbill showing total charges for hospital visits is mailed to the patient. When this method is used, the superbill is simply a means of sending a statement for hospital visits. It is not used in combination with the ledger card and daily log. (2) Other medical offices maintain a list showing the hospital admitting date of all patients. When a patient is discharged, total charges are recorded by the write-it-once method, using a superbill, ledger card, and daily log. The superbill is then mailed to the patient. (3) Using a third method, total charges made for hospital visits are recorded on the ledger card and daily log when the patient is discharged, and a routine statement is mailed during the billing cycle. No superbill is used. Figure 11-6 illustrates a superbill showing charges for hospital visits.

11.6 Recording Payments Received in the Mail

For checks, cash, or money orders received in the mail or brought in by a patient sometime after a service is performed, payments are posted only on the ledger card and the daily log. Follow the same procedure that was used for recording hospital charges. In Figure 11-5, the last three entries represent payments by mail or by delivery to the office.

174 The Modern Medical Office

Figure 11-6   Superbill Showing Charges for Hospital Care

```
| 8/10/- | Hospital Visits | 50.00 |         |            | 50.00   |          | C.R. Johnson | 112  |
|  DATE  |   DESCRIPTION   | CHARGE | PAYMENT | ADJUSTMENT | CURRENT | PREVIOUS |    NAME      | ACCT.|
|        |                 |        |         |            | BALANCE | BALANCE  |              | NUMBER|
```

This is your RECEIPT for this amount ▲   ▲ This is a STATEMENT of your account to date
ATTENDING PHYSICIAN'S STATEMENT   Patient *Chris Johnson*   Date of Service *8/8–8/9*

DIAGNOSES ARE ICD-9-CM CODED

☐ 412.0	Hypertension	☐ 227.3	Pituitary Neoplasm	☐ 242.2	Hyperthyroidism
☐ 786.50	Chest Pain	☐ 193.0	Thyroid Neoplasm	☐ 244	Hypothyroidism
☐ 413.9	Angina	☐ 490	Bronchitis	☐ 240.9	Goiter
☐ 428.0	C H F	☐ 324.0	Emphysema	☐ 242.3	Thyroid Nodule
☐ 425	Cardiomyopathy	☐ 493.9	Asthma	☐ 245.9	Thyroiditis
☐ 427.9	Cardiac Arrhythmia	☐ 079.9	Viral Syndrome	☐ 250.9	Diabetes
		☐ 558.9	Gastroenteritis		

OTHER DIAGNOSIS: _____

AMA CURRENT PROCEDURAL TERMINOLOGY - 4th EDITION

1. OFFICE VISITS — New / Estab-lished / FEE
   - Limited Visit ☐ 90010 ☐ 90050
   - Intermediate Visit ☐ 90015 ☐ 90060
   - Extended Visit ☐ 90017 ☐ 90070
   - Comprehensive Visit ☐ 90020 ☐ 90080

2. HOSPITAL SERVICES
   - Hospital: ☐ Metro ☐ _____
   - Admission/Hist.& Phy. ☐ 90220
   - Admit Date: ___198__
   - ICU Visits ☐ 90270
   - ___ visits @ ___ ea.
   - Hospital Visits ☒ 90260   *50.00*
   - *2* visits @ *25.00* ea.
   - Hospital Visit Limited ☐ 90250
   - ___ visits @ ___ ea.
   - (All Service Dates Below)
   - Date of Discharge _____ 198__

3. EMERGENCY ROOM
   - Brief Service   ☐ 90505 ☐ 90540
   - Extended Service ☐ 90517 ☐ 90570

4. HOSPITAL CONSULTATIONS
   - Limited   ☐ 90600
   - Intermediate ☐ 90605
   - Extended   ☐ 90610
   - Complex   ☐ 90620
   - Referring Physician _____

5. IMMUNIZATIONS-INJECTIONS
   - ☐ TET ☐ Flu ☐ Pneumovax   ☐ 90720
   - ☐ Testosterone
   - ☐ T-B Tine Test
   - ☐ _____

6. LABORATORY SERVICES — CPT — FEE
   - ☐ Chest Xray (PA)   71010
   - ☐ EKG   93000
   - ☐ CBC   85021
   - ☐ Urinalysis   81000
   - ☐ SMAC-20   80019
   - ☐ T-4   83440
   - ☐ Pap Smear   88100
   - ☐ Sed Rate   85650
   - ☐ Occult Blood Stool   82770
   - ☐ Glucose   82340
   - ☐ Cholesterol   82465
   - ☐ Protime   85610
   - ☐ Potassium   84132
   - ☐ WBC   84048
   - ☐ Hemoglobin   85018
   - ☐ Electrolytes   80003
   - ☐ Electrolytes, BUN, CR   80005
   - ☐ Thyroid Profile (T-7)   82756
   - ☐ TSH   84443
   - ☐ T3 RIA   84480
   - ☐ Thyroid Antimicro. Antibodies 85694
   - ☐ Prolactin   84146
   - ☐ Testosterone   84401
   - ☐ Glycohemoglobin   83020
   - ☐ SMAC - 20/T4   80019
   - ☐ Calcium   82310
   - ☐ Triglycerides   84478
   - ☐ Culture (Urine)   87086
   - ☐ Sensitivity (Urine)   87086
   - ☐ Culture (Throat Strep)   87060
   - ☐ Lateral Skull Film   70240
   - ☐ Blood Handling   99000
   - ☐ 24 Hour Urine For _____

7. OTHER SERVICES — FEE

TODAY'S FEES $ *50.00*

AUTHORIZATION TO PAY PHYSICIAN DIRECT
I hereby authorize payments directly to the undersigned Physician of the Medical Benefits, if any, otherwise payable to me for his services described above. I understand that I am responsible for the charges not covered by this authorization. I hereby authorize the undersigned Physician to release any medical information necessary to process this form.

Sign _____ Date _____
PATIENTS—Insurance claims handling procedures are explained on the reverse of the Pink Copy. KEEP THIS RECORD FOR INCOME TAX AND INSURANCE CLAIM FILING.

Return: ___ Days ___ Weeks ___ Mo.
Your Next Appointment _____ AM/PM
Day   Month   Date   Time

JOHN H. SPARKS, M.D.
8504 CAPRICORN DRIVE
ATLANTA, GA 30033-7775
(404) 555-0078

I.D. #20-83899022
S.S. #238-54-1345

Dates of Hospital Services
ICU Visits = 0
Hospital Visits = +
Limited = –

Mo ___ Yr ___ 1 2 3 4 5 6 7 *8* 9 10 11 12 13 14 15 16 17 18 19 20 21 22 23 24 25 26 27 28 29 30 31
Mo ___ Yr ___ 1 2 3 4 5 6 7 8 9 10 11 12 13 14 15 16 17 18 19 20 21 22 23 24 25 26 27 28 29 30 31

11.7   End-of-Day Financial Activities

At the end of each day after the last patient has been seen, each column of the daily log is totaled to show charges, credits, and total balance due. The summary of the daily log provides the physician with an understanding of the day's financial activities. Bank deposit totals should agree with the credits section of the daily log. Other summaries such as week-to-date, month-to-date, and year-to-date are prepared at this time. End-of-day summaries are shown in Figure 11-3.

Chapter 11—Accounting Procedures in the Medical Office **175**

11.8 Depositing the Day's Receipts

All cash, money orders, and checks are deposited in the bank each day. Money should not be kept in the office overnight. Follow these steps when making a bank deposit.

1. Count the currency and coins and record a total of each in the proper column of the bank deposit slip.

2. Write the American Banking Association (ABA) number which identifies the bank on which each check is drawn. This number is usually printed in the upper right corner of checks and is the top number of a two-part number divided by a horizontal line (see Figure 11-7). Write the amount of each check beside the ABA number. (Some people prefer to identify checks by the name of the person on whose account the check was drawn. Use the method your office prefers.)

Figure 11-7 Deposit Slip

DEPOSIT SLIP

BANK
DATE 6/14/--

RECEIPT NUMBER	ABA NO.	CASH		CHECKS	
		80	00		
1304	19-72			55	00
1308	6-21			15	
1309	11-14			15	00
1312	21-59			30	00

TOTAL CASH ▶ 80 00
TOTAL CHECKS ▶ 115 00
TOTAL DEPOSIT ▶ 195 00

DEPOSIT TO THE AMOUNT OF:
John H. Sparks, M.D.

3. Write the last name of the individual who signed each money order. Write the amount of each money order beside the individual's name.

4. Total the currency, coin, and checks column of the deposit slip. Check against the *Credits* section of the daily log. If adjustments are shown for any patients, subtract them from the credit section before a comparison is made with the deposit ticket. Adjustments are credits which do not involve an exchange of money. For example, an adjustment for an overcharge would not be included on the deposit slip. A deposit slip is shown in Figure 11-7. Compare it with the daily log in Figure 11-3.

12

Medical Billing and Collections

Billing and collection of patient accounts are important functions which require careful attention from the physician and the medical office staff. Since payment for medical services is the only revenue a medical office receives, the successful continuation of the practice depends on an efficient billing and collection process. Billing and collections may be handled internally by the medical office staff or externally by a private billing and collection service.

BILLING PATIENTS

12.1 External Billing

An outside billing service may be hired to manage patient accounts. The service maintains all ledger cards, posting debits and credits from copies of superbills which have been provided by the medical office. Monthly statements are prepared and mailed with a request that payment be returned to the billing service. Deposits are made directly to the physician's bank, and a report is prepared for the physician outlining all transactions. External billing services are valuable for practices which employ only a small clerical staff or which have a large number of patients. By placing the billing function with an outside agency, a major time-consuming clerical task is eliminated. The medical office employee acts as liaison between the billing service and the medical office and is responsible for coordinating their activities.

12.2 Internal Billing

Internal billing can be simple and fairly unsophisticated, with a copy of the ledger card serving as a statement. Or it can be highly complex, with a computer managing accounts and preparing statements. The size of the practice helps to determine the most efficient method of internal billing.

Superbill As Statement. The *superbill*, handed to each patient after charges for the visit have been calculated, is the first statement a patient receives. Since the best opportunity for collection is at the time of the visit, patients should be encouraged to pay when they are given the superbill. This also eliminates the time and cost of preparing and mailing a statement. Some medical offices accept major credit cards, as well as cash or checks, giving almost everyone a way to pay immediately.

Ledger Card As Statement. A copy of the ledger card mailed as a statement is a simple method of billing. Once each billing cycle, the ledger cards are copied, enclosed in window envelopes, and mailed to patients (see Section 6.34 for folding instructions). Since the ledger card shows all charges, credits, and adjustments, plus the patient's name and address, minimal time is spent on billing. To eliminate the need for checking each card for an outstanding balance, all ledger cards with outstanding balances can be coded with color strips visible at the top of the cards. When an account is paid in full, the color strip is removed. Another method is to store cards with outstanding balances in a special "Unpaid" section of the file which has been color coded (see Section 12.4).

Statement Form. In some medical offices, statement forms are prepared and mailed in window envelopes. The statement lists the patient's name and address, the date, a description of all services, and the medical fees. Preparing statements in this manner is a time-consuming task which is less efficient than mailing a copy of the ledger card, but a prepared statement looks better. A statement form is shown in Figure 12-1.

Computerized Statement. The most sophisticated billing is accomplished with a computer. Each billing cycle the medical office employee directs the computer to search through the files and print statements for patients with outstanding balances. The computer automatically ages accounts at the same time. For overdue accounts, a series of prewritten collection letters can be personalized and printed to remind patients that their payments are late (see Section 12.4). A computerized statement is shown in Figure 12-2.

Figure 12-1 Statement Form

John H. Sparks, M.D. 8504 Capricorn Drive Atlanta, GA 30033-7775		**STATEMENT** **FOR PROFESSIONAL** **SERVICES** **65342**		
Barbara Harper 802-B Georgetown Drive Atlanta, GA 30341-0796		**SERVICES FOR** Harper, Holly Lynn PAYMENTS RECEIVED AFTER Sept. 15 WILL BE APPLIED TO NEXT STATEMENT		

ENCLOSED $ _____

TO ASSURE PROPER CREDIT TO YOUR ACCOUNT, PLEASE DETACH AND RETURN THIS STUB

DESCRIPTION	PATIENT	DR CODE	DATE MO | DAY | YR	CHARGE	CREDIT
PREVIOUS BALANCE	65342		8/21/--	89.00	

PAY TO JOHN H. SPARKS, M.D.
POSTINGS ARE THROUGH 21ST OF AUGUST   89.00   PLEASE PAY ◀ THIS AMOUNT

180   The Modern Medical Office

Figure 12-2   Computerized Statement

```
                         BILLING INFORMATION
                         -------------------
                                                    Date:   04/25--


PATIENT NAME:   JOHNSON, HARRY-            ACCT#:   1-1-10
===============================================================================
    DATE        PROC. CODE    DESCRIPTION                         CHARGE
===============================================================================
 04/25/--         71021       X RAY CHEST AP/LAT                   35.00
 04/25/--         71456       DIGOXIN LEVEL                        57.00
 04/25/--         71457       ELECTROLYTES                         36.00
 04/25/--         PMT         Cash                                -75.00CR
                                                                 ----------
                                         TODAY'S BALANCE:         $53.00
                                         PREVIOUS BALANCE:       $153.00
                                         TOTAL BALANCE DUE:      $206.00

 -------------------------------------------------------------------------------
 DIAGNOSIS:   1)   RIGHT BUNDLE BRANCH BLOCK      5)
              2)   PVC'S                          6)
              3)                                  7)
              4)
 -------------------------------------------------------------------------------
 DATE OF FIRST SYMPTOM:                    04/22/--
 DATE FIRST CONSULTED FOR THIS CONDITION:  04/25/--

 REFERRING PHYSICIAN:  J. MONROE, M.D.   123 45TH ST.

===============================================================================
 ASSIGNMENT & RELEASE:    I hereby assign my insurance benefits to be
      paid directly to the undersigned physician.  I am financially
      responsible for noncovered services.  I also authorize the
      physician to release any information requested.


      Signed (Patient, or Parent if Minor):_____
                                     Date:_____
===============================================================================
                     Doctor's signature:_____
                                   Date:_____



 JOHN H. SPARKS, M.D.                   SS#:  238-54-1345
 8504 CAPRICORN DRIVE                   ID#:  20-83899022
 ATLANTA, GA  30033-7775
 PHONE: (404) 555-0078
```

12.3 Billing Periods

Monthly billing is a system in which all accounts are billed at the same time each month. *Cycle billing* is a system in which accounts are billed on a staggered schedule during the month.

Monthly Billing. When a monthly billing system is used, all statements are mailed near the end of the month, although they can be prepared earlier and stored until the mailing date. They also can be prepared in one or two days at the end of the month. When all statements are prepared just before the mailing date, other responsibilities may have to be neglected during this time. If several days pass between the preparation and mailing of statements, a message to "Disregard if payment has already been made" should be printed on the form.

Cycle Billing. When cycle billing is used, the alphabet is divided into sections, and patients are billed according to where the first letter of their last name falls in the alphabet. Each month, statements are prepared by the same schedule. A typical cycle billing schedule follows:

1. The alphabet is divided into four sections: *A-F, G-L, M-R, S-Z.*
2. Statements for patients whose last names begin with letters in the *A-F* section are prepared on Monday and mailed on Tuesday of Week 1.
3. Statements for patients whose last names begin with *G-L* are prepared on Monday and mailed on Tuesday of Week 2.
4. Statements for patients whose last names begin with *M-R* are prepared on Monday and mailed on Tuesday of Week 3.
5. Statements for patients whose last names begin with *S-Z* are prepared on Monday and mailed on Tuesday of Week 4.

COLLECTING FROM PATIENTS

Patients do not always pay their accounts on time; therefore, every medical office should have a collections policy. The medical office employee may handle collections, or overdue accounts can be given to a collection agency. Since the use of an agency is expensive, only large, long-past-due accounts should be given to them. Typically, unpaid accounts of more than $50 or $100 that are six months or more overdue are given to an agency, while the medical office employee handles routine collections. The final collection procedure is the filing of a lawsuit for nonpayment.

12.4 Aging Accounts

Aging accounts is a way of coding accounts according to the length of time they are unpaid. Strips of color coding can be attached to the ledger cards to show the age of an account, or the cards can be stored behind a color-coded divider in an "Unpaid" file. For example, a red code could be used for accounts one month overdue, a blue code for accounts two months overdue (see Figure 12-3). A written code such as "OD-2/14/--" can be written on the ledger card to indicate that an "overdue notice was sent on February 14, 19--." Aging systems differ

Figure 12-3 Color-Coded Ledger Card Indicating Overdue Balance

LEDGER SHEET
JOHN H. SPARKS, M.D.

Romero Sanchez 407
253-A Lost Creek Circle
Atlanta, GA 30033-2289

DATE	DESCRIPTION	CHARGE	CREDITS PAYMENT	ADJUSTMENT	CURRENT BALANCE
4/17/--	O.V., Xray	55.00	30.00		25.00
6/14/--	O.V., Lab	40.00	30.00		35.00

according to the type of patient being served. For example, a private patient's account is aged differently from that of a Medicare patient. In a computerized billing system, the accounts are automatically aged, and the aging code is shown on the computerized ledger card. A typical aging code for a private patient is given below:

1. S = Superbill given to patient at time of visit.
2. 1 = Itemized statement mailed after one month.
3. 2 = Itemized statement with overdue remark mailed after two months.
4. 3 = Letter saying, "We have not received payment for your account" after three months.
5. 4 = Letter saying, "Your account is overdue" after four months.
6. 5 = Letter saying, "Your account will be turned over to a collector" after five months.
7. 6 = Letter saying, "Your account was turned over to the collection agency" after six months.
8. 7 = Collection agency attemps to collect.
9. 8 = Lawsuit filed.

12.5 The Collection Letter Series

Lack of payment usually is not considered serious until after 60 days. When the patient has not responded to either the statement or the "Overdue" notice at the end of 60 days, the series of collection letters begins. A typical collection series is shown in Figures 12-4, 12-5, 12-6, and 12-7.

12.6 Collections When Insurance Is Involved

Many patients have private medical plans, such as Blue Cross/Blue Shield, or qualify for government insurance, such as Medicare or Medicaid. While some medical offices will not file and follow up insurance claim forms for patients, other medical offices do handle these forms. When agencies do not pay in full or question or deny a claim, the medical office assistant determines what the problem is and notifies the patient. Figures 12-8 to 12-13 concern insurance claims.

12.7 Truth in Lending

The Truth in Lending Act requires a physician to outline clearly the terms of any payment plan for fees that are financed by the physician. Figure 12-14, page 189, confirms a Truth in Lending agreement with a patient.

Figure 12-4 First Collection Letter

```
                JOHN H. SPARKS, M.D.
                8504 CAPRICORN DRIVE
                 ATLANTA, GA 30033-7775
                     (404) 555-0078


June 27, 19--


Mr. Nathaniel Alexander
1438 Ashbury Court
Decatur, GA  30033-1667

Dear Mr. Alexander:

Your account with our office has been neglected and is
now seriously past due. Please make some attempt to
reduce your balance of $93.50 immediately.

Please call us if you have any questions about your
account.

Sincerely,

Mary Sue Brandon
Mary Sue Brandon
Accounts Manager
```

Figure 12-5 Second Collection Letter

```
                JOHN H. SPARKS, M.D.
                8504 CAPRICORN DRIVE
                 ATLANTA, GA 30033-7775
                     (404) 555-0078


July 26, 19--


Mr. Nathaniel Alexander
1438 Ashbury Court
Decatur, GA  30033-1667

Dear Mr. Alexander:

Your account balance of $93.50 remains overdue after
four months. We expected that you would pay your
account within a reasonable amount of time after treat-
ment at our office.

A reasonable amount of time has passed, and we cannot
continue to keep your unpaid account on our books.

Please send payment immediately or call me with a
reason why you cannot pay. If we do not hear from you,
we will be forced to take further action.

Sincerely,

Mary Sue Brandon
Mary Sue Brandon
Accounts Manager
```

Chapter 12—Medical Billing and Collections   **185**

Figure 12-6 Third Collection Letter

JOHN H. SPARKS, M.D.
8504 CAPRICORN DRIVE
ATLANTA, GA 30033-7775
(404) 555-0078

August 28, 19--

Mr. Nathaniel Alexander
1438 Ashbury Court
Decatur, GA 30033-1667

Dear Mr. Alexander:

You must contact me personally within 14 days of receipt of this letter, or your account balance of $93.50 will be turned over to the Georgia Adjustment Bureau for collection.

If you will call me, I will be happy to arrange a payment plan that is suitable for you as well as for us.

Sincerely,

Mary Sue Brandon

Mary Sue Brandon
Accounts Manager

Figure 12-7 Fourth Collection Letter

JOHN H. SPARKS, M.D.
8504 CAPRICORN DRIVE
ATLANTA, GA 30033-7775
(404) 555-0078

August 15, 19--

CERTIFIED MAIL

Mr. Nathaniel Alexander
1438 Ashbury Court
Decatur, GA 30033-1667

Dear Mr. Alexander:

This letter is our final attempt to collect your account, which is six months past due. Several statements and letters have been sent to you, but you have not responded. The balance of $93.50 remains outstanding.

Your account is being turned over to the Georgia Adjustment Bureau which will pursue whatever legal means is necessary to collect this debt. If you contact me within seven days, we will remove your account from the adjustment bureau. This will protect your credit rating.

Sincerely,

Mary Sue Brandon

Mary Sue Brandon
Accounts Manager

186 The Modern Medical Office

JOHN H. SPARKS, M.D.
8504 CAPRICORN DRIVE
ATLANTA, GA 30033-7775
(404) 555-0078

June 18, 19--

Mrs. Rachael Manfried
623-A, Building One
Colony Square
Fairburn, GA 30213-1818

Dear Mrs. Manfried:

We have received a notice from Medicaid that no payment will be made on your account with Dr. Sparks. Therefore, you are responsible for the medical fees.

Please make full payment of your $128 outstanding balance within the next thirty days, or contact me so that we can arrange a payment plan.

Sincerely,

Mary Sue Brandon
Mary Sue Brandon
Accounts Manager

Figure 12-8 Letter to Patient Regarding Medicaid

JOHN H. SPARKS, M.D.
8504 CAPRICORN DRIVE
ATLANTA, GA 30033-7775
(404) 555-0078

June 19, 19--

Miss Veronica Crawford
7845 Bridgewater Lane
Decatur, GA 30033-1265

Dear Miss Crawford:

In order to file an insurance claim for the services Dr. Sparks performed for you on June 8, some information is needed for the insurance company. Please answer the questions listed below and return this letter to our office within ten days.

1. Medicare Number
2. Medicaid Number
3. Blue Cross/Blue Shield Group Number
4. Blue Cross/Blue Shield Contract Number
5. Name of Blue Cross/Blue Shield Subscriber
6. Other Insurance Name
7. Other Insurance Policy Number
8. Other Insurance Company Name and Address

Thank you, Miss Crawford, for your help.

Sincerely,

Mary Sue Brandon
Mary Sue Brandon
Accounts Manager

Figure 12-9 Letter Asking for Insurance Information

Chapter 12—Medical Billing and Collections 187

Figure 12-10 Letter Informing Patient of Insurance Rejection

JOHN H. SPARKS, M.D.
8504 CAPRICORN DRIVE
ATLANTA, GA 30033-7775
(404) 555-0078

December 7, 19--

Mr. Lee Chung
3459 Jackson Lane
College Park, GA 30354-0871

Dear Mr. Chung:

We have received a notice from your insurance company that no benefits are payable under your policy for Dr. Sparks's services. Therefore, you will be responsible for full payment of your account which has an outstanding balance of $345.

If you are unable to make payment immediately, please contact our office so that together we may set up a reasonable payment schedule.

Sincerely,

Mary Sue Brandon
Mary Sue Brandon
Accounts Manager

Figure 12-11 Letter Seeking Information from Insurance Company

JOHN H. SPARKS, M.D.
8504 CAPRICORN DRIVE
ATLANTA, GA 30033-7775
(404) 555-0078

June 17, 19--

Blue Cross/Blue Shield of Georgia
428 Peachtree Street
Atlanta, GA 30333-2021

Ladies and Gentlemen:

    Patient Name: Mary Anderson
    Subscriber Name: Robert Anderson
    Group Number: 34-621-81
    Contract Number: 4-621-81
    Date of Service: 5/14/--
    Date Claim Submitted: 5/17/--

We have not received payment for the above patient's claim for an appendectomy performed on May 14, 19--. A copy of the claim form we filed with your agency is enclosed.

Please check the status of this claim and notify the patient and our office of your findings.

Sincerely,

Mary Sue Brandon
Mary Sue Brandon
Accounts Manager

enclosure

Figure 12-12 Letter to Government Agency Regarding Nonpayment

```
            JOHN H. SPARKS, M.D.
           8504 CAPRICORN DRIVE
           ATLANTA, GA 30033-7775
                (404) 555-0078
```

June 7, 19--

Medicare
675 Peachtree Street
Atlanta, GA 30303-1720

Ladies and Gentlemen:

Patient Name: Alice Naylor
Patient Address: 128 Highland Avenue
                 Atlanta, GA 30308-7730
Medicare Number: 423-3456-23a

A medicare form was filed with your agency on April 6, 19--, for payment of Ms. Naylor's claim. Since that time, several requests have been made for payment, but we have received no correspondence from your office. A copy of Ms. Naylor's claim form is attached.

Please check your files and notify us of your findings. If you are unable to make payment on these charges or if you need additional information, please contact me.

Sincerely,

Mary Sue Brandon

Mary Sue Brandon
Accounts Manager

enclosure

Figure 12-13 Workers' Compensation Letter to Employer

```
            JOHN H. SPARKS, M.D.
           8504 CAPRICORN DRIVE
           ATLANTA, GA 30033-7775
                (404) 555-0078
```

March 15, 19--

Mr. Oswald Bosch
Acme, Ltd.
340 Industrial Park Drive
Enigma, GA 31749-1941

Dear Mr. Bosch:

Your insurance company has not paid its claim on behalf of your employee, Helen Spada. Please contact your carrier to determine the status of this claim; inform us of your findings. Failure to do so will force us to bill your employee for the balance.

Sincerely,

Mary Sue Brandon

Mary Sue Brandon
Accounts Manager

Chapter 12—Medical Billing and Collections **189**

Figure 12-14 Truth in Lending Disclosure

JOHN H. SPARKS, M.D.
8504 CAPRICORN DRIVE
ATLANTA, GA 30033-7775
(404) 555-0078

June 18, 19--

Mr. Blake Merritt
456 Carver Lane
Decatur, GA 30033-4970

Dear Mr. Merritt:

As agreed in our conversation today, special arrangements have been made for the payment of your account. Please sign the enclosed form and return it to our office.

Sincerely,

Mary Sue Brandon
Mary Sue Brandon
Accounts Manager

enclosure

Figure 12-14 (continued)

JOHN H. SPARKS, M.D.
8504 CAPRICORN DRIVE
ATLANTA, GA 30033-7775
(404) 555-0078

TRUTH IN LENDING

This disclosure is made in compliance with the Truth of Lending Act.

Margaret Merritt, Child   Blake Merritt
Patient's Name   Guarantor's Name

                                             456 Carver Lane
8974   Atlanta, GA 30032-4428
Patient's Number   Address

1. Cash Price Medical Fee $800
2. Less Cash Down Payment   200
3. Unpaid Balance of Cash Price   600
4. Amount Financed   600
5. Finance Charge   60
6. Total of Payments (3 plus 4)   660
7. Deferred Payment Price   660
8. Annual Percentage Rate   10%

The total of payments is payable to Dr. John H. Sparks at the address shown above in 12 installments of $55, the first installment being payable August 1, 19--, and all subsequent payments being due on the first day of each month.

_____   _____
Date   Guarantor's Signature

13

Word Processing in the Medical Office

13.1 Word Processing—What Is It?

Word processing is a system used to process written communications through the use of modern equipment, greater employee specialization, and an increase in standardized procedures.

Word Processing Definition

Begin With	Add	Result
Traditional system for processing written medical communications	New, modern equipment and/or Greater employee specialization and/or Increase in standardized procedures	WORD PROCESSING, a system to process written medical office communications

Medical offices that would like to benefit from the increased efficiency and reduced costs of word processing do not have to use all the word processing components. A small medical office may wish to add some of the modern, automatic equipment. A large medical office may wish to employ all the word processing components to revamp a system for processing written communications.

13.2 Word Processing—Why?

Because governments require more reports, because medical offices have expanded, and because there is a greater need for medical offices to protect against legal action, the volume of paperwork in today's medical offices has increased. The combination of increased paperwork, higher production costs, and fewer medical office workers has resulted in decreased office productivity. Concern over this situation has led many medical offices to focus on ways to increase the efficiency of originating, producing and revising, duplicating, distributing, and storing written medical communications.

Modern office equipment may provide part of the solution. Electronic typewriters, stand-alone word processors, personal computers, and computer scopes connected to a larger mainframe computer use magnetic tape, magnetic cards, cassette tapes, floppy disks, hard disks, or memory for storage and type at speeds ranging from 150 to over 600 words per minute. Dictation methods include the use of desk microphones, telephones in the office or any other location, and portable dictation units small enough to slip into a pocket.

While some medical offices do improve efficiency through the simple addition of modern equipment, other medical offices find it beneficial to also incorporate greater employee specialization and an increase in standardized procedures. Thus, the benefits of word processing include the following:

- Handwritten input or dictation (personal or machine) can be handled quickly.

- Production increases because interruptions from nontyping duties are minimized.

- Corrections and revisions are made easily and quickly.

- Even work loads result from the assignment of medical clerical support on the basis of need.

- High morale and low employee turnover result from adequate supervision and evaluation as well as increased opportunities for career advancement.

13.3 Word Processing—How Does It Work?

In all medical offices the flow of written communications proceeds in five stages: originating, producing and revising, duplicating, distributing, and storing. Table 13-1 shows each of these stages and how they take place in the *traditional* medical office.

Table 13-1
Flow of Written Communications in the Traditional Medical Office

Stages	Methods and Equipment Used
Originating	Longhand Dictation to Medical Secretary
Producing and Revising	Electric Typewriter Self-correcting Typewriter
Duplicating	Carbon Copies Stencil Duplication Offset Duplication Copying Machines
Distributing	Interoffice Mail U.S. Postal Service Alternative Mail Systems
Storing	Traditional Files Microfilm Microfiche

Word processing provides additional options for each stage in the processing of written communications.

An understanding of some specialized terminology will assist the medical office worker in understanding the capabilities of word processing systems.

Electronic Typewriter: Electric typewriters with limited memory and a few word processing features.

Stand-Alone (Dedicated) Word Processors: Fully equipped automatic typewriters with software designed for heavy-use word processing. These systems use magnetic cards, diskettes, or hard disks for storage. Increased memory and complete text-editing features are included.

Personal Computer Hardware: Personal computer equipment, including the display screen, the keyboard, the printer, and the drives.

Personal Computer Software: Specialized programs which provide instructions to the computer for particular applications such as word processing, spreadsheets, data management, graphics, job-specific education, personal financial management, communications, and entertainment.

Transcription: The process of taking input (usually in person or by machine dictation) and keyboarding it into mailable form.

Word Processing Menus: The array of choices provided by any word processing software program once it is activated. For example, an "opening menu" might provide a choice of opening an existing file for revision; opening a new file to create a document; renaming a file; copying, printing, or deleting a file; or asking for "help" (additional assistance). A subsequent menu within a file would provide choices for setting margins; moving, inserting, or deleting characters, words, lines, or tabs; saving the file; or moving to other menus with additional, more complex choices.

Mail Merge: This software allows the creation of personalized form letters, mailing labels, invoices, and other documents. It merges text with variable data base information, such as names and addresses, to produce a final merged letter.

Spreadsheet: Spreadsheets—automated ledger sheets such as *Lotus 1 2 3* (Lotus Development Corp.)—are known as the "number crunchers" of software. A spreadsheet program allows the computer to provide a blank electronic blackboard of rows and columns. Spreadsheet medical programs such as the *P.M.S. Medical Billing System* can handle and track up to 10,000 active accounts.

Data Base Systems: Programs that act like electronic filing cabinets, organizing data into files, records, and fields. They are excellent for recording, sorting, updating, and classifying data. One medical office example is *Nutrient Analysis,* which can handle a data base of up to 10,000 foods. Once a patient's sex and age group are entered, this program determines recommended intake of cholesterol and 26 nutrients. It can be used to analyze food items and meals, as well as daily, weekly, and monthly menus.

Telecommunications Software: A computer program that lets your computer, with a modem hookup through a telephone line, communicate with another computer at the other end of the line. A good example in the medical office is the phonogram cardiogram. A patient's EKG is transmitted via the office computer to another computer for preliminary interpretation (using data such as age, weight, sex, and medications) and for a stand-by specialist review. Some equipment prints results directly on the EKG itself; others require a phone call to get results. In all cases a cardiologist, or other medical doctor, must interpret the final results.

Optical Scanners: Devices that can scan or "read" material into the computer without rekeying. At present, optical scanners have limited reading abilities. In the future, however, all typewritten material (and perhaps handwritten information as well) will be scanned via a light pen and entered into the computer automatically.

Networking: The process of hooking computer to computer (personal computer to mainframe computer, personal computer to stand-alone word processor) via hard-wiring (actual wires between personal computer and mainframe) or through telephone lines using a modem. Networking permits the transfer of documents between users and allows for central storage of computer records.

Facsimile Machines: Copying machines that electronically send and receive typed pages, photos, and graphs via telephone lines; thus producing instant copies in remote locations.

Integrated Applications Program: Software that combines many separate uses into one integrated program. For example, *Lotus Symphony* (Lotus Development Corp.) combines spreadsheet, data base, and word processing programs and provides easy transfer of data between each application.

13.4 Originating

Origination can occur at most levels within a medical organization. The following are the originating processes used with word processing.

Originating Stage Using Word Processing

Traditional Methods	Additional Methods Used with Word Processing
Longhand	Machine Dictation Using:
Face-to-Face Dictation	Desktop Unit
	Portable Unit
	Centralized System with Microphones or Telephones

While longhand and face-to-face dictation to a medical secretary are still used with a word processing system, most origination takes place using machine dictation. Since physicians were among the first major users of machine dictation, most medical offices are already using one component of word processing. Desktop dictation units, portable dictation units, or centralized dictation systems are used. The desktop or portable units commonly record dictation on cassette tapes; centralized dictation systems use continuous loop tapes to record dictation via a desktop microphone or over regular medical office or hospital telephone lines.

Word processing can speed the originating process by standardizing dictation procedures. These procedures provide information for the medical transcriber on the type of dictation (letter, memo, etc.), the urgency of each item dictated, the number of copies needed, and special instructions on desired format, addresses, and closing requirements. Originators are urged to organize their thoughts before beginning medical dictation. Successful dictation requires practice and feedback. This includes feedback to the originators on how dictation can be improved and feedback to the transcriber on how subsequent medical transcription can be improved.

Another process of origination within word processing systems involves the use of *standardized letters* (also called *form letters*). In many medical offices, there are situations that call for the repeated use of basically the same letter. Follow-up letters on delinquent medical accounts are one example of repeat medical correspondence; another might be a letter to another physician requesting transfer of medical records for a new patient. Rather than write an original letter for each of these similar occurrences, many medical offices draft well-written standardized letters to be used with variable information inserted by the originator. Figures 13-1 and 13-2 are examples of both a standardized letter and the variable information that an originator would provide.

13.5 Producing and Revising

The second stage in the written communications process—producing and revising—involves taking the input from the originator; transforming it into a typed, mailable medical transcript; and making subsequent corrections or revisions. Revisions or corrections to work returned to the originator from word processing should be indicated using standard proofreader's marks (see Figure 13-3). Once revised copy has been returned, the originator need only proofread corrections indicated, since other text should remain the same.

It is during the producing and revising stage that the most impact is felt from the addition of word processing. The following is a summary of the producing and revising processes used in word processing.

Producing and Revising Stage Using Word Processing

Traditional Methods	**Additional Methods Used with Word Processing**
Electric Typewriter	Transcribing Machines
Self-Correcting Typewriter	Electronic Typewriters
	Dedicated Word Processors
	Personal Computers
	Optical Scanners
	Networking

Dedicated word processors (defined in Section 13.3) come with word processing programs. While these word processing programs can, in some instances, be upgraded with additional features, their main purpose and design is for word processing.

196 The Modern Medical Office

Figure 13-1 Standardized Medical Letter

```
                    ──────────────── Ⓐ
                    ────────────────
                    ────────────────
     Ⓑ ────────────
Dear ──────── Ⓒ ────────, ──── Ⓓ ────
When you visited the office on ─────────, you will
recall that a pap smear was taken as part of your normal
medical checkup.

The results of this test are back from our laboratory
analysis, and the findings are:
              ──────── Ⓔ ────────

These results require Ⓕ ──────────────────
                       ──────────────────
Please call the office at 274-4483 if you have any questions
regarding these test results.
                                    Sincerely

                                    Alberta Goodman, D.O.

mos
cc: Ⓖ ──────────
```

Figure 13-2 Variable Information for Standardized Letter

Tampa Medical Center, P.A.

Standardized Letter Request

This request is for standardized letter # **43**

Letter Title **Pap Results**

Requestor **Alberta Goodman**

Department **OB/Gyn**

Date of Request **2/9/-**

Please print variable information:

A **Current date**

B **Mrs. Elsa Agramonte**
   4725 N.W. 2nd Court, Plantation, FL 33318-6509

C Dear **Mrs. Agramonte**

D **January 4, 1985**

E **normal**

F **no immediate action; checkup in one year**

G **Dr. Louis Berger**

H

I

J

SPECIAL INSTRUCTIONS
Send Dr. Berger a copy of lab report

Figure 13-3 Proofreader's Marks

PROOFREADER'S MARKS

Mark	Meaning	Example	Result
∧	insert copy	Please send to me.	Please send it to me.
⌒	close up	to day	today
#	add space	maybe	may be
∪	transpose	It cuold be moved easily.	It could be easily moved.
/ or lc	lowercase	She WILL take care of the Deed.	She will take care of the deed.
ℓ	delete	our WP manager	our manager
ℓ (with close up)	delete and close up	forgotttten	forgotten
/	replace	of rome	on time
⊙	insert period	E M Myers	E. M. Myers
___	underline	NCAS Newsletter	NCAS Newsletter
≡	capitalize	wp center	WP center
sp	spell out	5 documents	five documents
¶	new paragraph	Indent each paragraph five spaces. ¶ Type the writer's name in caps.	Indent each paragraph five spaces. Type the writer's name in caps.
stet or	let it stand; ignore the correction	Take some time for yourself.	Take some time for yourself.
∧	insert punctuation	May 12 19--	May 12, 19--
═	straighten line	Even this out.	Even this out.
⌐	move right	This is wrong.	This is wrong.
⌐	move left	This is also wrong.	This is also wrong.
⌒	move copy as indicated	Place the word on the next line.	Place the word on the next line.
SS	single-space	36 Luther Street Oneonta, NY 13820-6601 Dear Ms. Kent	36 Luther Street Oneonta, NY 13820-6601 Dear Ms. Kent
DS	double-space		
TS	triple-space	1,123,465 3,649,000	1,123,465 3,649,000

The cost, size, and complexity of these dedicated word processors created a class of equipment known as electronic typewriters (defined in Section 13.3). Electronic typewriters are generally used by offices with a limited need for fully equipped word processing units. Many of these electronic typewriters can be upgraded with additional features, even to the extent that they finally become dedicated word processors. However, the cost of such upgrading, compared to the word processing capability ultimately achieved, needs to be considered when making such a purchase.

Personal computer hardware and computer software with medical office applications (defined in Section 13.3) are available. One of the most frequently used software applications within a medical office is word processing. Most of the medical-specific software programs, however, concentrate on billing, appointment scheduling, and keeping track of group practices.

Word processing on the personal computer is possible with word processing software or an integrated applications program. Word processing software is comprised of menu choices which can perform the following functions: text editing (corrections, additions, deletions, and movement of text); margin, type size, and spacing specifications; underlining, boldfacing, and footnoting adjustments during printing; file management; and special features and writing aids such as spelling check, mail merge, and math capability. While the first word processing programs such as *Wordstar* (Micropro International Corp.) and *Microsoft Word* (Microsoft Corp.) were written independently of dedicated word processing programs, more recent entries to the word processing software market include programs that emulate dedicated word processor functions (*Display Write* [IBM Corp], *Office Writer* [Wang Systems]), thus eliminating the need for operator retraining.

Integrated applications programs (defined in Section 13.3) contain word processing and at least one other application within the same software program. For example, the *Lotus Symphony* (Lotus Development Corp.) program contains five functions: word processing, communications with other personal computers, a spreadsheet, data base manager, and graphics.

The personal computer allows the sharing of information between various data and word processing files. The use of an integrated application program makes such sharing easier and faster. Patient test results, for example, could be included in a letter to a consulting physician without having to rekey all the results. Rather, the computer goes to the file containing the test results, extracts them, and inserts them into the letter.

Proceed slowly and carefully when making changes involving word processing. Hardware and software must be evaluated together before a purchase is made, and dealer support and training should be an important component in purchasing decisions. Several medical office employees should be trained on any new system in case of illness or turnover of medical office personnel.

Optical scanners and networking (defined in Section 13.3) should be considered in planning for word processing. They will allow for rapid exchange of information between users and between systems.

13.6 Duplicating

The following is a summary of the duplicating processes used with word processing.

Duplicating Stage Using Word Processing

Traditional Methods	Additional Methods Used with Word Processing
Carbon Copies	Automatic Typewriter Originals
Stencil Duplication	Letter Quality or Matrix Printers
Offset Duplication	Phototypesetting
Copy Machines	Facsimile Machines
	Laser Printers
	Networking

As indicated above, the four duplicating processes used in the traditional office can also be used in a word processing system. Copying machines, however, are probably the most commonly used in both. With word processing, an unlimited number of automatic typewriter originals of any page desired can be printed quickly. Phototypesetting can be done with letter-quality printers and with word processing software designed to justify right margins.

Facsimile machines (defined in Section 13.3) quickly send and receive typed pages via telephone lines. Printers attached to a network (defined in Section 13.3) receive medical correspondence directly from a dedicated word processor or personal computer along with instructions for the number of copies required. Networking also allows copy duplication on the screen of any equipment in the same network.

13.7 Distributing

The following is a summary of the distributing processes used with word processing.

Distributing Stage Using Word Processing

Traditional Methods	Additional Methods Used with Word Processing
Interoffice Mail	Teletypewriters
U.S. Postal Service	Facsimile Machines
Alternative Mail Systems	Networking
	Satellite Communications
	Modem

Mail systems within the traditional office are discussed in Sections 6.28-6.37.

Teletypewriters send and receive typed messages via telephone lines using Telex or TWX. Facsimile machines reproduce both typed documents and pictures in distant locations as described in Section 13.3.

Networking provides the capability for electronic mail with instant distribution. Growing satellite communications and microwave towers allow messages to be beamed throughout the world and connect one network to another for distribution. Satellite and microwave communications are faster and cheaper than using telephone lines.

13.8 Storing

The following is a summary of the storing processes used with word processing.

Storing Stage Using Word Processing

Traditional Methods	Additional Methods Used with Word Processing
Traditional Files	Floppy Disks
Microfilm	Fixed/Hard Disks
Microfiche	Shared Logic Storage
	Mainframe Computers

Traditional medical filing systems are discussed in Chapter 7.

Microfilm and microfiche are not new to the office. However, with a word processing system, some businesses are now using micrographics (microfilm and microfiche) to store active records. Such a system can reduce office storage requirements by more than 90 percent. Dedicated word processors and personal computers use floppy disks to store medical correspondence. Some personal computers come with a hard disk, thus allowing the rapid storage of and access to huge quantities of data. Networking provides access to centralized storage via shared logic systems or mainframe computers, thus centralizing records and providing high-speed access. Rising costs of medical office space make these systems advantageous.

13.9 Word Processing—The Future

Whether or not word processing can add to the efficiency of any medical office is a question for careful study. Medical office requirements, costs, and personnel must be given careful consideration in any decision-making process. Each word processing component and the organization of these components should be reviewed. Visits to other word processing centers are useful. One thing is certain—technology will continue to provide more ways to handle written communications in the medical office. Whether or not you are using word processing in your medical office today, you should make an effort to keep current with this rapidly changing field.

14

The Computer in the Medical Office

Computers, which were originally used by hospitals for billing and administration, have found their way into private medical practices. They are revolutionizing the medical office by handling routine clerical and accounting tasks which were once time-consuming responsibilities of the medical office employee. Use of a computer usually results in increased collections, reduced errors, and a savings in time.

COMPUTERIZED ACCOUNTING

A computer can handle medical accounting activities in a fraction of the time required for pegboard accounting. Because the human element is reduced, fewer errors result from a computerized system. A large number of accounting programs are available in many medical specialty areas, and most can be customized to meet the needs of an individual practice. While each program has specialized features, most are similar and have the same basic features as a pegboard system.

14.1 Account Management

Management of patient accounts is an effective use of a computer. On the first visit to the medical office a new patient completes an information form that asks for personal information, the name of the patient's insurance company, and the name of the guarantor of the account (see Section 5.1). The medical office employee keyboards this information into the computer in about one minute's time. Debits, credits, and adjustments from superbills can then be entered as they occur over the following weeks or months. The computer automatically creates and updates the ledger card, adds new names to the list of patients and the daily log, and manipulates the data to produce insurance forms, statements, a list of checks received each day, and deposit slips. The computer automatically ages accounts at each billing cycle (see Section 12.4). A typical first visit information screen is shown in Figure 14-1.

Figure 14-1   Computer Information Screen

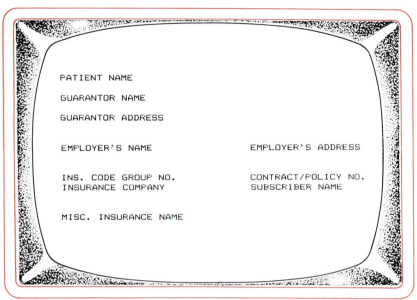

Account management software automatically matches procedures to procedure codes, diagnoses to diagnosis codes, and calculates charges for services. When a procedure code is entered, the computer responds by automatically adding a description of the procedure and a charge to the patient's ledger. When a diagnosis code is entered, the computer responds by automatically adding diagnosis information to insurance forms.

The following description of the features of *The Physician's Office Computer,* a software package for doctors' offices, outlines some of the features a medical office staff could expect from a computer system.

14.2   Computerized Superbill

The superbill, as described in Section 11.1, can also be used in a computerized accounting system. When the patient or nurse returns the superbill to the receptionist, charges are entered into the computer and automatically posted to the ledger card. A hard copy (paper copy) is printed for the patient's records. A computerized superbill is shown in Figure 14-2.

Figure 14-2 Computerized Superbill

```
                                                                                    Aging Information
JOHN H. SPARKS, M.D.        STATEMENT DATE   08/29/--
8504 CAPRICORN DRIVE        PATIENT NUMBER   113
ATLANTA, GA  30033-7775     PREVIOUS BALANCE -->       $0.00
                                                                OFFICE PHONE: (404) 555-0078
   DATE    | CODE  |     DESCRIPTION          |  AMOUNT
  02/12/-- | 00000 | BALANCE FORWARD          |   23.00         STATEMENT DATE   08/29/--
  02/16/-- | 71020 | CHEST X RAY, 2 VIEWS     |   40.00
  03/14/-- | 80010 | URINALYSIS               |   20.00         CURRENT           0.00
  04/22/-- | 85022 | CBC                      |   12.50         OVER 30-DAYS     52.00
  06/13/-- | 90220 | INIT. HOSP. EXAM, EXTENSIVE | 75.00        OVER 60-DAYS     75.00
  07/05/-- | 93040 | RHYTHM STRIP             |   17.00         OVER 90-DAYS      1.85
  07/26/-- | 93000 | ELECTROCARDIOGRAM        |   35.00         BALANCE DUE   $128.85
  08/29/83 | PMT   | PERSONAL CK              |  -93.65CR
                                                                 THANK YOU FOR YOUR PAYMENT.

                       BALANCE DUE:              $128.85
                                                                 113
  OFFICE CLOSED SEPTEMBER 5TH     JOHN H. SPARKS, M.D.          LINDA S. HAYLEY
                                  8504 CAPRICORN DRIVE          532 5TH STREET
  NEW CHARGES HAVE BEEN SENT      ATLANTA, GA  30033-7775       ATLANTA, GA  30033-2385
  TO YOUR INSURANCE CARRIER(S).
```

Procedure Codes — Procedures

14.3 Computerized Patient Ledger

A computerized patient ledger contains personal information about a patient, including the patient's name, address, responsible parties, insurance carriers, employer's phone number, plus a listing of all procedures and procedure codes and all charges, payments, and adjustments. Some computerized ledgers provide additional information. Most can be customized to meet the special needs of an individual medical office. They may be viewed on the computer screen or printed as needed. Figure 14-3 shows a patient ledger which was produced by a computer. Notice the description of the procedures and the charges which were automatically included after procedure codes were entered.

14.4 Daily Log

The daily log is generated from information entered on each patient's superbill. At the end of each day, the computer automatically produces a daily log which reports payments, charges, and adjustments by patient name and number. These reports usually show the total number of patients seen each day, plus the day's total billings, collections, and adjustments. A wide variety of other "canned" statistical information is available, or the daily log can be customized to the financial reporting needs of an individual practice. The daily log can be developed for a single physican or for an entire practice on command. A daily log produced by computer is shown in Figure 14-4.

Chapter 14—The Computer in the Medical Office 205

Figure 14-3 Computerized Patient Ledger Card

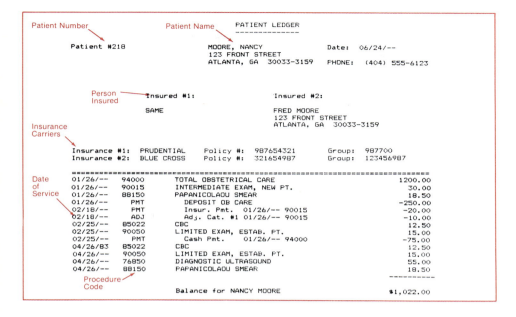

Figure 14-4 Daily Log Produced by Computer

```
                    DAILY JOURNAL OF CHARGES AND PAYMENTS
                                 05/20/--

PAT NO    NAME              DATE      PROCEDURE                              N-SVS    CHARGE      PAYMENT DR
======================================================================================================
1001      ALLAN, ROBERT     0502--    32000  THORACOCENTESIS                   8    $ 640.00    $    0.00
1001                        0520--    36800  UDALL CATHETER INSERTION          1    $ 110.00    $   50.00
1001                        0520--    71020  CHEST X RAY, 2 VIEWS              1    $  30.00    $    5.00
1001                        0501--    83498  HYDROXYPOGESTERONE-17             4    $ 120.00    $   10.00
1001                        0520--    83020  HEMOGLOBIN                        1    $  20.00    $    0.00
1001                        0520--    90450  NURSING HOME VIST, LTD SER. (@2   1    $  20.00    $    0.00
1001                        0520--    999.2  ADJ 90450   830520  830520        0    $ -20.00    $    0.00
1001                        0520--    999.2  ADJ 830520  830520  36800         0    $-110.00    $  -50.00
1023      BROWN, NAOMI      0520--    82910  EXECUTIVE PROFILE-31 TEST         1    $  54.00    $   24.00
1023                        0504--    90080  ANNUAL RENAL CHECK UP             4    $ 300.00    $   50.00
1023                        0520--    999.2  ADJ 830504  830512  90080         0    $-300.00    $  -50.00
1030      CARDEN, ANNETTE L 0520--    92950  CARDIOPULMONARY RESUSCITATION     1    $ 100.00    $    0.00
1030                        0520--    93510  FEMORAL CATHETER                  1    $  50.00    $   25.00
1030                        0520--    81000  URINALYSIS                        1    $   9.75    $    0.00

MODE       NUMBER       TOTAL
=====================================
0  CASH          9    $    0.00
1  CHECK         1    $    5.00
2  MONEY ORDER   1    $   10.00
3  VISA          1    $    0.00
4  MASTERCARD    2    $   49.00
5  INSURANCE     0    $    0.00
6  ADJUSTMENT    0    $    0.00

                                          TOTALS
          CHARGES $1023.75    PAYMENTS $  64.00    ADJUSTMENTS $  0.00    NO OF PATIENTS  3
```

14.5 Insurance Forms

Private insurance forms as well as Medicare, Medicaid, and Workers' Compensation insurance claim forms can be printed from the computer system. The forms show the diagnosis and diagnosis code, the procedure and procedure code, the charges, plus other information. Insurance forms can be printed individually or in bulk on a daily, weekly, or monthly basis at the rate of about four per minute. The computer will print two insurance forms automatically if the patient has two policies. (The policy names and numbers are entered from the information form at the time of the patient's first visit.) When a Workers' Compensation claim is made, a computer system can produce the physician's first report of work injury, as well as the Attending Physician's Report. In medical offices which do not complete insurance forms for patients, the computer generates a detailed superbill for the patient to attach to the insurance form. Figure 14-5 illustrates an insurance form generated by computer.

14.6 Billing Statements

On command, a medical office computer prints billing statements showing detailed charges, payments, and adjustments. Finance charges are added automatically, and the patient's account is aged at the same time. The computer prints the appropriate aging reminder or letter to accompany the statement (see Section 12.4). Figure 14-6, page 208, illustrates a statement produced by computer.

14.7 Cash and Check Register

A computer system can produce a register of cash and checks that includes the necessary American Banking Association numbers. The report may be attached to a bank deposit slip without further manual work. A check register is shown in Figure 14-7, page 208.

14.8 Automatic Cross-Posting

A computer system can track the application of fees for multiple-physician practices when the physicians provide service to each other's patients. This can be provided as a daily, weekly, or monthly transaction report.

14.9 Aged-Accounts Receivables Reports

A computer system can age accounts according to a variety of criteria, including past due, zero balance, or credit balance accounts by age category or by insurance carrier. For example, a report might include all of Dr. Sparks's Medicare accounts over 60 days past due. An aged-accounts receivables report is shown in Figure 14-8, page 209.

Chapter 14—The Computer in the Medical Office

Figure 14-5 Insurance Form Generated by Computer

PRUDENTIAL
4123 PRUDENTIAL PLAZA
ATLANTA, GA 30033-1775

HEALTH INSURANCE CLAIM FORM
READ INSTRUCTIONS BEFORE COMPLETING OR SIGNING THIS FORM

MEDICAID ☐   MEDICARE ☐   CHAMPUS ☐   OTHER ☒

FORM APPROVED
OMB NO. 66-R0012

PATIENT & INSURED (SUBSCRIBER) INFORMATION   EMPLOYER: SELF

1. PATIENT'S NAME (First name, middle initial, last name)
MOORE, NANCY

2. PATIENT'S DATE OF BIRTH
09 | 12 | 52

3. INSURED'S NAME (First name, middle initial, last name)
SELF (PATIENT)

4. PATIENT'S ADDRESS (Street, city, state, ZIP code)
123 FRONT STREET
ATLANTA, GA 30033-3159
TELEPHONE NO

5. PATIENT'S SEX
MALE ☐   FEMALE ☒

6. INSURED'S I.D. MEDICARE AND/OR MEDICAID NO. (Include any letters)
987654321

7. PATIENT'S RELATIONSHIP TO INSURED
SELF ☒   SPOUSE ☐   CHILD ☐   OTHER ☐

8. INSURED'S GROUP NO. (Or Group Name)
987700

9. OTHER HEALTH INSURANCE COVERAGE - Enter Name of Policyholder and Plan Name and Address and Policy or Medical Assistance Number
BLUE CROSS
FRED MOORE
321654987

10. WAS CONDITION RELATED TO
A. PATIENT'S EMPLOYMENT
YES ☐   NO ☒
B. ACCIDENT
AUTO ☐   OTHER ☐

11. INSURED'S ADDRESS (Street, city, state, ZIP code)
SAME AS ABOVE

12. PATIENT'S OR AUTHORIZED PERSON'S SIGNATURE (Read back before signing)
I Authorize the Release of any Medical Information Necessary to Process this Claim and Request Payment of MEDICARE Benefits Either to Myself or to the Party Who Accepts Assignment Below
SIGNED SIGNATURE ON FILE   DATE

13. I AUTHORIZE PAYMENT OF MEDICAL BENEFITS TO UNDERSIGNED PHYSICIAN OR SUPPLIER FOR SERVICE DESCRIBED BELOW
SIGNATURE ON FILE
SIGNED (Insured or Authorized Person)

PHYSICIAN OR SUPPLIER INFORMATION

14. DATE OF ILLNESS (FIRST SYMPTOM) OR INJURY (ACCIDENT) OR PREGNANCY (LMP)
12/02/--

15. DATE FIRST CONSULTED YOU FOR THIS CONDITION
01/25/--

16. HAS PATIENT EVER HAD SAME OR SIMILAR SYMPTOMS?
YES ☐   NO ☒

16a. IF AN EMERGENCY CHECK HERE ☐

17. DATE PATIENT ABLE TO RETURN TO WORK

18. DATES OF TOTAL DISABILITY
FROM   THROUGH

DATES OF PARTIAL DISABILITY
FROM   THROUGH

19. NAME OF REFERRING PHYSICIAN OR OTHER SOURCE (e.g., public health agency)
NORMAN JOHNSON, M.D.   ATLANTA, GA 30033-1115

20. FOR SERVICES RELATED TO HOSPITALIZATION GIVE HOSPITALIZATION DATES
ADMITTED   DISCHARGED

21. NAME & ADDRESS OF FACILITY WHERE SERVICES RENDERED (If other than home or office)
MEDICAL LAB, INC.   456 TESTTUBE ROAD

22. WAS LABORATORY WORK PERFORMED OUTSIDE YOUR OFFICE?
YES ☒   NO ☐   CHARGES $0.00

23. DIAGNOSIS OR NATURE OF ILLNESS OR INJURY. RELATE DIAGNOSIS TO PROCEDURE IN COLUMN D BY REFERENCE NUMBERS 1,2,3, ETC. OR DX CODE
1. NORMAL PREGNANCY
2. TRICHOMONAL VAGINITIS
3.
4.

B. EPSDT   YES ☐   NO ☐
FAMILY PLANNING   YES ☐   NO ☐

PRIOR AUTHORIZATION NO. _____

24. A DATE OF SERVICE	B PLACE OF SERVICE	C. FULLY DESCRIBE PROCEDURES, MEDICAL SERVICES OR SUPPLIES FURNISHED FOR EACH DATE GIVEN PROCEDURE CODE (IDENTIFY)	(EXPLAIN UNUSUAL SERVICES OR CIRCUMSTANCES)	D DIAGNOSIS CODE	E CHARGES	F DAYS OR UNITS	G T.O.S.	H. LEAVE BLANK
06/26/--	3	85022	CBC	1	12 50			
06/26/--	3	90050	LIMITED EXAM. ESTAB.	1,2	15 00			
06/26/--	3	76850	DIAGNOSTIC ULTRASOUND	1	55 00			
06/26/--	3	88150	PAPANICOLAOU SMEAR	2	18 50			

25. SIGNATURE OF PHYSICIAN OR SUPPLIER
(I certify that the statements on the reverse apply to this bill and are made a part hereof.)
SIGNED *John H. Sparks, M.D.* DATE 6/16/--

26. ACCEPT ASSIGNMENT (GOVERNMENT CLAIMS ONLY) (SEE BACK)
YES ☐   NO ☐

27. TOTAL CHARGE $101 00
28. AMOUNT PAID -0-
29. BALANCE DUE $101 00

30. YOUR SOCIAL SECURITY NO
123-46-6844

31. PHYSICIAN'S OR SUPPLIER'S NAME, ADDRESS, ZIP CODE & TELEPHONE NO
JOHN H. SPARKS, M.D.
8504 CAPRICORN DRIVE
ATLANTA, GA 30033-7775
(404) 555-0078

32. YOUR PATIENT'S ACCOUNT NO
2

33. YOUR EMPLOYER I.D. NO
95-32414

I.D. NO.

*PLACE OF SERVICE AND TYPE OF SERVICE (T.O.S.) CODES ON THE BACK
REMARKS

APPROVED BY AMA COUNCIL ON MEDICAL SERVICE 5-80
APPROVED BY THE HEALTH CARE
FINANCING ADMINISTRATION & CHAMPUS

Form **AMA-OP-407**
Form **HCFA-1500 (4-80)**
Form **CHAMPUS-501**

Figure 14-6 Statement Produced by Computer

```
                    BILLING INFORMATION

                                          Date:   04/25/--

PATIENT NAME: JOHNSON, HARRY-          ACCT#: 1-1-10

  DATE       PROC. CODE    DESCRIPTION                         CHARGE

04/25/--     71021         X RAY CHEST AP/LAT                   35.00
04/25/--     71456         DIGOXIN LEVEL                        57.00
04/25/--     71457         ELECTROLYTES                         36.00
04/25/--     PMT           Cash                                -75.00CR

                                   TODAY'S BALANCE:            $53.00
                                   PREVIOUS BALANCE:          $153.00
                                   TOTAL BALANCE DUE:         $206.00

DIAGNOSIS:   1)  RIGHT BUNDLE BRANCH BLOCK       5)
             2)  PVC'S                           6)
             3)                                  7)
             4)

DATE OF FIRST SYMPTOM:                 04/22/--
DATE FIRST CONSULTED FOR THIS CONDITION:  04/25/--

REFERRING PHYSICIAN:  J. MONROE, M.D.   123 45TH ST.

ASSIGNMENT & RELEASE:   I hereby assign my insurance benefits to be
paid directly to the undersigned physician.  I am financially
responsible for noncovered services.  I also authorize the
physician to release any information requested.

    Signed (Patient, or Parent if Minor):_____
                                         Date:_____

    Doctor's signature:_____
                  Date:_____


JOHN H. SPARKS, M.D.                      SS#:  239-54-1345
8504 CAPRICORN DRIVE                      ID#:  20-83899022
ATLANTA GA 30033-7775
PHONE: (404) 555-0078
```

Figure 14-7 Check Register

```
                 JOHN H. SPARKS, M.D.

                 CHECK REGISTER FOR:  06/17/--

TOTAL NUMBER OF CHECKS:                              5

TOTAL AMOUNT OF CHECKS:                       $2194.50

TOTAL CASH RECEIVED:                             $0.00

TOTAL DEPOSIT                                 $2194.50


                       CHECKS RECEIVED

CK. NO.    ABA NO.       AMOUNT     PATIENT NAME      PATIENT NO.

1) 9087654              86.00       WOLFF, DEAN        02-1-102
2) 3425678900          978.00       JONES, HARRY       02-1-105
3) 7681980            1023.50       BALSAM, REBECCA    02-1-95
4) 76543869             67.00       ISAACS, KAREN      02-1-90
5) 483                  40.00       HYCHE, FEARL       02-1-100
```

Chapter 14—The Computer in the Medical Office

Figure 14-8 Aged-Accounts Receivables Report

```
                              AGED-ACCOUNTS RECEIVABLES AS OF 08/10/--

USER SELECTED VARIABLES:   BALANCE DUE: BALANCE OWING    AGING: CURRENT AND OVER
                           INSURANCE:   All              DOCTOR: JOHN H. SPARKS, M.D.                    PAGE 1
```

NUMBER	PATIENT NAME	BAL. DUE	CURRENT	31-60	61-90	91-120	>120	LAST PMT.	AMOUNT	FORM
2-1-23	JOHNSON, ROSIE PHONE: 559-5623 MC 897654 8769543	197.50	----	197.50	----	----	----	----	----	
2-1-25	KELLY, YOLANDA PHONE: 924-7387 BC 9368356 DS123 MC 987645	162.50	110.00	52.50	----	----	----	07/30/--	40.00	Ins.
2-1-40	DAVIS, RAY PHONE: 456-9909 BC 2345 4567 MC 123456789	751.50	751.50	----	----	----	----	07/28/--	15.00	Cash
2-1-41	HEATH, PERCY PHONE: 721-5858 BC 9987654 AS123 MC 9876543	292.00	257.00	----	35.00	----	----	07/29/--	50.00	Cash
2-1-42	WOODWARD, GREG PHONE: 252-4569 PR 54361892 LK212 MC 894765	197.50	197.50	----	----	----	----	08/04/--	85.00	M-cal
2-1-43	DANIELS, BRUCE PHONE 714 853-7569 213 545-9612 AE 472351 AK1578 PR 54896 T6J147	227.50	110.00	50.00	67.50	----	----	08/04/--	35.00	Cash

2-1-44	MAJORS, BRAD
	PHONE 213 466-6251
	AE 987654 AE 82 J
	MC 12345678
	FAMILY ACCOUNT MEMBERS:
	  MAJORS, BETTY 2-1-47
	  MAJORS, JANET 2-1-45
	  MAJORS, BRAD JR. 2-1-48
		1108.50	1108.50	----	----	----	----	08/04/--	30.00	M-cal

14.10 Production Report Analysis

A computer system can automatically produce a report of all procedures performed by each doctor or group of doctors, showing the month-to-date and year-to-date frequency and the dollar volume produced.

14.11 Doctors' Billings and Collections Reports

A computer system can maintain a daily, monthly, and yearly total of billings and collections.

DATA BASE MANAGEMENT

Data base management is a system whereby large quantities of data can be accessed, searched, sorted, and arranged very rapidly by computer. A data base management system can greatly reduce the time spent in file management.

14.12 Computerized Data Base Management

With a computer, it is easy to develop a data base of patients, drugs, supplies, diseases, or any other category of information the physician wishes to monitor. After the data has been entered, it can be sorted and reported according to name, patient number, ZIP Code, date of service, insurance company name, procedure, diagnosis, medication, or any other classification. For example, if a drug is recalled, a search through the patient data base can produce a list of all patients to whom the drug was given. If a research project is undertaken about an illness, the data base can be searched for the names of all patients who have the illness. Figure 14-9 is a partial list of Dr. Sparks's patients whose names start with *A*. Figure 14-10 is a partial list of Dr. Sparks's patients who have ZIP Codes that begin with 30033. Each list was generated by commanding the computer to sort through all patient names and print according to alphabet and ZIP Code.

14.13 Recall and Reminder Notices

Data base management allows the computer to produce follow-up appointment dates and check-up dates. Reminder notices can be stored in the patient's file and printed automatically as the computer searches the data base for names of patients needing appointments.

Figure 14-9   List of Patients Whose Names Begin with "A"

LAST NAME	FIRST NAME	PATIENT NUMBER	CITY	STATE	ZIP
ADAMS	ALICIA	907	ATLANTA	GEORGIA	30303-6754
AFTON	ROOSEVELT	236	FAIRFIELD	GEORGIA	30345-1151
ALLISON	FAY	453	DECATUR	GEORGIA	30033-7997
ARMER	WILLIAM	634	ATLANTA	GEORGIA	30303-8562
AWORK	MONICA	821	DECATUR	GEORGIA	30033-2658

Figure 14-10   List of Patients According to ZIP Code

ZIP CODE	LAST NAME	FIRST NAME	PATIENT NUMBER	CITY	STATE
30033-7997	ALLISON	FAY	453	DECATUR	GEORGIA
30033-2658	AWORK	MONICA	821	DECATUR	GEORGIA
30033-5897	BAKER	MARTIN	367	DECATUR	GEORGIA
30033-9976	CANTRELL	ANGELIA	654	DECATUR	GEORGIA

14.14   Labels

Labels can be produced from the patient list. The labels can be used for mailings, charts, a telephone card file, specimens, and other purposes.

14.15   Research

Patient information stored in a data base can be used to develop research reports. For example, a study of an allergy requires the names of all patients who are treated for the allergy, the medications prescribed, reactions to the medication, and success of the treatment. From this and other information, the physician may be able to draw conclusions and make recommendations about treatment.

14.16   Electronic Appointment Scheduling

Appointments can be made, changed, cancelled, confirmed, and printed from the computer. Each doctor within the system can have individual appointment slots, free times, and days off. The computer manages all appointments, searching through the internal appointment book for available openings. A daily list of appointments can be generated from the electronic appointment schedule.

HARDWARE

Hardware refers to the computer and related peripheral equipment such as printers, disk drives, and monitors or screens. While hardware is basic to a computer system, the hardware should be purchased only after the software has been selected.

14.17   Types of Computers

Computers fall into three major categories: (1) mainframe computers, (2) minicomputers, and (3) microcomputers. *Mainframe computers* are large, highly sophisticated computers capable of manipulating and storing large quantities of data. Hospitals frequently use mainframe computers for storing medical records. *Minicomputers* look like mainframe computers and are also able to manipulate and store large quantities of data, but the memory capacity of a minicomputer is not as great as that of a mainframe computer. Large medical centers are likely to use a minicomputer. *Microcomputers,* or personal computers, are sometimes called desktop computers because they are small enough to fit on the top of a desk. Microcomputers today are so sophisticated that their capability is as great as the mainframe computers of the 1950s. Small and average-sized medical practices are most likely to use a microcomputer. Popular microcomputers which run medical software are available from Texas Instruments, Apple Computer, IBM, Radio Shack, and other manufacturers.

14.18   Memory Capacity

A computer's memory must be large enough to support the software you wish to use and to manipulate the data you enter. A software vendor is able to say how much memory each program requires. A good rule of thumb is to buy a computer with at least 256K of temporary memory; however, the capability to expand the computer's memory in the future is more important than the amount of memory purchased initially. As computer software becomes more sophisticated, greater memory capacity will be required.

14.19 Configuring Computer Equipment

Configuring computer equipment is the combining of pieces of computer equipment and the physical arrangement of the pieces. For example, a medical office might have a configuration of two microcomputers, one in the physician's office and one in a medical office employee's work area, plus one matrix printer in the physician's office and one letter-quality printer in the employee's office. The equipment is configured so that both the office staff and the physician can use it efficiently.

14.20 Floppy Diskettes and Hard Disks

Floppy diskettes are small magnetic disks on which computer information is stored. Diskettes are available in several sizes: 8 inch, 5 1/4 inch, and 3 1/2 inch. The type of computer you have determines the size of diskette you use. Called "floppy" because they bend, diskettes can hold a limited number of files. They are satisfactory for storing the number of records a small medical practice of one or two physicians might have, but they are not satisfactory for storing a large number of records.

Hard disks are capable of storing large quantities of information and can be used satisfactorily for storage of many medical records. Additional hard disks can be added to some computer systems, increasing the amount of storage capability.

SOFTWARE

Software is the program which tells the computer what to do. Programs are available for a variety of purposes, including accounting, word processing, graphics, data base management, education, and others. The quality of the software determines how easily and successfully a task is handled.

14.21 Importance of Proper Selection of Software

Finding good software should be the primary concern when purchasing computers. A great deal of time should be spent previewing several software packages before the purchase of any software is made. Since all software does not run on all computers, the computer to be used depends on its compatibility with the software selected. Some medical offices make the mistake of first purchasing a computer and then purchasing software which runs on the particular brand of computer. This usually results in frustration for the office staff due to the inability of the computer to perform all the necessary tasks.

14.22 Checklist for Purchase of Computer Software

The Medical Office Computer Shopper's Checklist provides a comprehensive guide for purchasing computer software for the medical office.

1. How easy is it to use the system?
2. How many systems are currently in the field?
3. How long has the company been in business?
4. Will they provide names of current users? (If not, forget about them. Be sure to check out the referrals. They will tell you a lot more than the salesperson.)
5. Will they train your office staff as much as necessary, and how much after-sale support will they guarantee?
6. How much training will be necessary before the system may be operated by your staff, and is this training included in the cost of the system?
7. Can you understand what the salesperson is showing you? (If not, the office staff will have more trouble.)
8. Can you enter your own data into the system and see the reports, or are you only seeing a prearranged demonstration?
9. Will they provide on-site maintenance and what is the cost?
10. What about software updates? (Every system needs occasional changes.)
11. Do they offer one-step service or will you have to deal with two, three, or more vendors to maintain the computer? (With more than one vendor, it is possible that no one will accept responsibilty for a problem.)
12. How thorough and well-written is the owner's manual?
13. What enhancements are currently in the works?
14. What are each of the reports the computer supplies?
15. How are you protected in case of power failure or system malfunction?
16. Are hard-copy printouts readily available for all transactions and other valuable information?
17. Who makes the hardware and how reliable is it? (Check with current users about this.)
18. How many patients will the system handle?
19. How many doctors will the system handle?

20. How many transactions will the system handle daily?

21. How many patients may be maintained with complete ledgers for one year?

22. Does the system maintain a permanent record of all patients, or are they removed every time their balance is 0?

23. How well-supported is the system by other hardware and software vendors?

24. Is it a hard disk or floppy disk system?

25. Can the system be easily and cost effectively expanded and upgraded?

14.23 Graphics

Graphics software allows a computer to produce images on the screen or on paper. Graphics software is important to a medical office because it allows the author of a research document to develop bar charts, pie charts, and line graphs to include in the document.

14.24 Word Processing

Medical reports and correspondence can be produced efficiently and accurately with a word processing software package. Documents can be edited and printed as often as necessary. (see Sections 13.4-13.6).

14.25 Electronic Communication

By adding communication capability to a computer, a medical office is able to communicate via telephone lines with computers in other parts of the city or the country. Transplant donors and recipients, for example, are usually located through computer hookups at different hospitals. Communication capability also allows the medical office to subscribe to private medical, financial, and other data base services. A physician, for example, might subscribe to the Dow Jones Financial Service for stock information or to a medical data base for information about diseases.

COMPUTERS AND CONFIDENTIALITY

Computer technology, with its opportunities for record keeping, represents a potential problem for patient confidentiality. Data bases of patient records in private offices and hospitals can be accessed by individuals with a knowledge of computers. Confidentiality of computerized patient records is a problem which every medical office should address.

14.26 AMA Position on Computer Security

Computer security is an important issue addressed by the American Medical Association. The Association has adopted guidelines for patient records in computer data bases. With the permission of the AMA, the guidelines are given below.

1. Confidential medical information entered into the computer should be verified as to the authenticity of its source.

2. The patient and the physician should be advised about the existence of computerized data bases in which medical information concerning the patient is stored. Such information should be communicated to the physician and patient prior to the physician's release of the medical information. All individuals and organizations with access to the computerized data bank (and the level of access permitted) should be specifically identified in advance.

3. The physician and patient should be notified of the distribution of all reports reflecting identifiable patient data prior to distribution of the reports by the computer facility. There should be approval by the physician and patient prior to the release of patient-identifiable data to individuals or organizations external to the medical care environment. Such information should not be released without the express permission of the physician and the patient.

4. The dissemination of confidential medical data should be limited to only those individuals or agencies with a bona fide use for the data. Release of confidential medical information from the data base should be confined to the specific purpose for which the information is requested and limited to the specific time frame requested. All such organizations or individuals should be advised that authorized release of data to them does not authorize their further release of the data to additional individuals or organizations.

5. Procedures for adding to or changing data on the computerized data base should indicate individuals authorized to make changes, time period in which changes take place, and those individuals who will be informed about changes in the data from the medical records.

6. Procedures for purging the computerized data base of archaic or inaccurate data should be established and the patient and physician should be notified before and after the data has been purged. There should be no commingling of a physician's computerized patient records with those of other computer bureau clients. In addition, procedures should be developed to protect against inadvertently mixing of individual reports or segments thereof.

7. The computerized medical data base should be on-line to the computer terminal only when authorized computer programs requiring the medical data are being used. Individuals and organizations external to the clinical facility should not be provided on-line access to a computerized data base containing identifiable data from medical records concerning patients.

8. Security:

   A. Stringent security procedures for entry into the immediate environment in which the computerized medical data base is stored and/or processed or for otherwise having access to confidential medical information should be developed and strictly enforced so as to prevent access to the computer facility by unauthorized personnel. Personnel audit procedures should be developed to establish a record in the event of unauthorized disclosure of medical data. A roster of past and present service bureau personnel with specified levels of access to the medical data base should be maintained. Specific administrative sanctions should exist to prevent employee breaches of confidentiality and security procedures.

   B. All terminated or former employees in the data processing environment should have no access to data from the medical records concerning patients.

   C. Involuntarily terminated employees working in the data processing environment in which data from medical records are processed should be removed from the computerized media data environment.

   D. Upon termination of a computer service bureau's services for a physician, those computer files maintained for the physician should be physically turned over to the physician or destroyed (erased). In the event of file erasure, the computer service bureau should verify in writing to the physician that the erasure has taken place.

MEDICAL SOFTWARE REFERENCES

Medacs Medical Accounting System, Advanced Computer Systems, 3131 South Dixie Drive, Dayton, OH 45439

Medical Office Management, CMA, Microcomputer Division, 55722 Santa Fe Trail, Yucca Valley, CA 92284

MEDI-LOG, Colwell Systems, Inc., 201 Kenyon Road, Champaign, IL 61820

Medirec, CMA, Microcomputer Division, 55722 Santa Fe Trail, Yucca Valley, CA 92284

Physician's Office Computer, Professional Systems Corporation, 1240 Kona Drive, Compton, CA 90202

Sandman Software Services, Inc., P. O. Box 65, 2500 Highway 79S, Guntersville, AL

15

Parts of Speech

The skills medical employers most want are basic academic skills—the ability to read, write, communicate, compute, and think logically. This unit will focus on language usage by providing guidelines for identifying and using parts of speech.

You should be familiar with the major parts of speech—nouns, pronouns, adjectives, verbs, adverbs, prepositions, and conjunctions. These are the categories we use to refer to the part each word plays within a sentence. Sometimes the same word can be used as a noun and a verb. Notice the use of *mix* in the following sentences:

Noun: The *mix* of ingredients was just right.
Verb: Please *mix* the ingredients thoroughly.

When a word plays a different role in a sentence, it often changes form:

Noun: gratitude
Verb: gratify
Adjective: gratifying

In the dictionary, the pronunciation guide immediately follows the word, and that is followed by the word's part of speech.

15.1 Nouns

The most frequently used words are *nouns*. Nouns identify persons, places, things, or ideas.

Persons: Ms. Cristina Mateo, technicians, Patrick
Places: Miami, Henry Ford Hospital, laboratory
Things: cystoscope, acid, heart
Ideas: ethics, morality, justice

Common Nouns and Proper Nouns. There are two kinds of nouns: *common nouns*, which are generic names for persons, places, things, or ideas and are not capitalized; and *proper nouns,* which refer to a particular person, place, thing, or idea and are always capitalized.

Common Nouns

doctor
hospital
organization
speech

Proper Nouns

Dr. Anabel Farinas
Mt. Sinai Hospital
American Medical Association
State of the Nation Address

The plural forms of nouns are generally formed by adding *s:*

Singular

nurse
operating room
desk

Plural

nurses
operating rooms
desks

Some nouns, however, are made plural according to different rules:

Singular

knife
bench
child

Plural

knives
benches
children

Always consult the dictionary if you are unsure of the correct plural form of any noun.

Compound Nouns. A *compound noun* is formed when two or more words are combined and used as a single noun. Compound nouns are sometimes hyphenated:

father-in-law
self-defense

sometimes combined and written as one word:

pacemaker
downtown
overhead

sometimes written as two or more words:

operating room
attorney general

Since compound nouns are written in a variety of ways, it is always a good idea to consult a dictionary for the exact spelling of these nouns. If the compound word is not in the dictionary, it should be written as two separate words. When a compound noun is part of a company name, however, always follow the style shown on the company's letterhead.

15.2 Pronouns

Pronouns are "shorthand" for nouns. When a noun has been identified, or is understood, the shorter pronoun is used in place of the noun.

The physical therapists agreed that *they* wanted John as *their* vice-president.

Using the pronoun sounds better than always repeating the noun:

The physical therapists agreed that the physical therapists wanted John as the physical therapists' vice-president.

The pronouns *they* and *their* replaced the noun *therapists*. The noun which a pronoun replaces is called its *antecedent,* meaning "coming before." The antecedents are shown in all capital letters in the following examples:

Dr. Kenneth Stringer read the laboratory REPORTS, put *them* in an ENVELOPE, and slid *it* into his briefcase.
The board EXAMINATIONS are given quarterly, *they* last two days, and *they* are known to be very difficult.

Indefinite Pronouns. When pronouns do not refer to a specific person, place, or thing (no antecedent), they are known as *indefinite pronouns*.

Singular: another, anybody, anyone, anything, each, either, every, everybody, everyone, everything, many a, neither, no one, nobody, nothing, one, somebody, someone, something
Plural: both, few, many, several, others
Singular and Plural: all, none, some

Personal Pronouns. *Personal pronouns* are those pronouns that change form to indicate person. You can write or speak from three points of view. In *first person* you talk about yourself or about a group of which you are a member. In *second person* you talk about the person(s) you are speaking to, and in *third person* you speak of anyone or anything else.

First Person Singular

I, my, mine, me

First Person Plural

we, our, ours

This is *my* uniform.
Our laboratory work reveals elevated blood glucose.

Second Person Singular

you, your, yours

Second Person Plural

you, your, yours

Your check-in at the hospital is scheduled for noon.
You all have a chance to aid in the diagnosis.

Third Person Singular

he, his, him, she, her, hers, it, its

Third Person Plural

they, their, theirs, them

Her lab coat is red.
Pass out the medication to *them,* please.

Compound Pronouns. When *-self* (singular) or *-selves* (plural) is added to a pronoun, a *compound* or *reflexive* pronoun is created.

First Person: myself, ourselves
Second Person: yourself, yourselves
Third Person: himself, herself, themselves, itself

Case. Not only do pronouns change form to indicate person, they also change form to indicate their function in a sentence. This pronoun function is identified as one of three cases: *nominative, objective, and possessive.*

The nominative case of the pronoun is used when the pronoun is the subject of the sentence (what the sentence is about) or when the pronoun is the complement of the sentence (completing, or adding meaning to, the verb).

Nominative Prounouns—I, we, you, he, she, it, they, who, that, whoever, which, what

As the subject:

She (not her) has been elected president of the Michigan Osteopathic Physicians.
They (not them) are reviewing the X rays.

As the complement:

The one with the infectious disease might be *he* (not him).
Dr. Carlyle said he was the one *who* (not whom) took the medical history.

The objective case of the pronoun is used when the pronoun is the object of the verb (the action of the verb is directed at the pronoun), when the pronoun is the object of a preposition (part of a prepositional phrase), or when the pronoun is the subject or object of an infinitive (*to* plus a verb).

Objective Pronouns—me, us, you, him, her, it, them, whom, whomever, that, which, what

As the object of the verb:

Ed gave Suzanne and *me* (not I) help on the patient billing.

As the object of a preposition:

The ampicillin was prescribed for *him* (not he).

As the subject or object of an infinitive verb:

The doctor asked *her* (not she) to apply. (*Her* is the subject of *to apply*.)
Did the doctors ask Lila Mae to consult *them* (not they)? (*Them* is the object of *to consult*.)

The possessive case of the pronoun is used when the pronoun indicates possession. When the possessive pronoun precedes the noun, use *my, our, your, his, her, its,* or *their*. When the possessive pronoun is separated from the noun it modifies (describes), use *mine, ours, yours, his, hers, its,* or *theirs*.

My instruments are right here. (preceding noun)
The instruments on the cart are *mine*. (separated from noun)

Sometimes possessive pronouns are confused with similar-sounding contractions (shortened words where the apostrophe indicates omitted letters). Avoid this mistake.

Possessive Pronouns	Contractions
whose	who's (who is)
your	you're (you are)
its	it's (it is)
their	they're (they are)
theirs	there's (there is)

15.3 Adjectives

Adjectives are words used to describe nouns and pronouns. Adjectives tell you which one, how many, what kind, or what size.

The *little* spot on the *patient's* X ray was discovered by the *alert* radiologist. *Thirteen* nurses arrived at the *square* building in the middle of the *Calle Ocho Festival*.

A noun preceded by *the* indicates a specific person, place, or thing, so *the* is referred to as a *definite adjective* or *definite article*. Use of *a* or *an* indicates no specific person, place, or thing; thus, it is referred to as an *indefinite adjective* or *article*. Remember to use *an* before all words beginning with a vowel (*a, e, i, o,* and short *u*) and also before all words that sound like they begin with a vowel (*hour*). With all other words, use *a*.

Definite: *The* patient came in for several diagnostic tests.
Indefinite: *An* individual must study hard in order to pass nurses' training.
A local dilatation on the walls of *an* artery is known as *an* aneurysm.

Pronouns become adjectives when they are used to modify nouns:

Her fever was higher than *his* fever.
This research paper on bacteria has many examples of *those* errors.

15.4 Verbs

The most common sentence errors involve the misuse of verbs. Therefore, an understanding of the way verbs are used within a sentence can improve your ability to communicate effectively and accurately.

In order for a sentence to be complete, it must have both a subject and a verb. While a noun or pronoun can be the subject of a sentence (the doer of the action) or the object of the sentence (the receiver of the action), it is the verb that indicates the action. The verb indicates what the subject does or is, or what is happening to it.

Verbs make statements:

The lab report *is* now complete.
Dr. Patrick Gettings *will be* our next doctor.

Verbs give commands:

Answer the call, please.
Remain in the clinic until I return.

Verbs ask questions:

Who *will attend* the medical convention?
Is this your nurses' pin?

Active or Passive Voice. Sentences in which the subject performs the action of the verb are said to be in the *active voice*.

Dr. Mateo diagnosed the illness.
The insurance agent mailed the pictures of the accident.

The subjects—*Dr. Mateo* and the insurance *agent*—performed the action indicated by the verb.

If the subject of the sentence is being acted upon, the sentence is said to be in the *passive voice*.

The blood was delivered by courier.
Mario was operated on last week.

The subjects—*blood* and *Mario*—received the action indicated by the verb.

Agreement of Subject and Verb. One of the most common grammatical problems is finding the right form of the verb to go with the subject of the sentence. The subject and verb in the same sentence should *agree,* meaning that a singular subject requires a singular verb and a plural subject requires a plural verb.

Singular Subject, Singular Verb: The *report is* (not are) almost complete.
 He is (not are) the new nurse.
Plural Subject, Plural Verb: Three *women were* (not was) in the lobby.
 The *doctors are* (not is) taking golf lessons.

A compound subject requires a plural verb.

Compound Subject, Plural Verb: *Bill and Mary have been* (not has been) treated for poison ivy.

When a group is the subject of a sentence, and the group acts collectively with a single purpose, a singular verb is used.

Group Acting Together, Singular Verb: The *committee recommends* (not recommend) a complete reorganization of the Vicente Medical Center.

When the members of a group act independently, as many different persons completing the same action, a plural verb is used.

Group Acting Independently/Plural Verb: The *staff are* (not is) at their desks.

Verb Tense. Verbs also tell time. The *tense* of the verb indicates the time of the event. Refer to Table 15-1, page 226, for assistance with each of the six verb tenses: past, past perfect, present, present perfect, future, and future perfect. Depending upon the "time" of what you are writing about, select the appropriate verb tense.

Helping Verbs. *Helping verbs* are joined to other verbs to indicate voice or tense. Common helping verbs include:

are	have
can	have been
can be	is
can have	may
could	may be
could be	may have
could have	may have been
could have been	might
did	might be
do	might have
had	might have been
had been	must
has	must be
has been	must have

must have been	will
shall	will be
shall be	will have
shall have	will have been
shall have been	would
should	would be
should be	would have
should have	would have been
should have been	

Regular and Irregular Verbs. All *regular verbs* form the various tenses in the same way as the example shown in Table 15-1. *Irregular verbs,* however, form the present, past, future, and past participle verb forms in a variety of unexpected ways. Always consult your dictionary for assistance, since the principal parts of all irregular verbs are listed. If such parts are not shown, the verb is regular.

Common Irregular Verbs

Present	Past	Past Participle
am, are, is	was, were	been
become	became	become
begin	began	begun
bring	brought	brought
buy	bought	bought
come	came	come
do	did	done
drive	drove	driven
fall	fell	fallen
get	got	got
give	gave	given
go	went	gone
grow	grew	grown
know	knew	known
leave	left	left
lay	laid	laid (to place)
lie	lay	lain (to rest)
make	made	made
pay	paid	paid
run	ran	run
see	saw	seen
spring	sprang	sprung
take	took	taken
write	wrote	written

Table 15-1
Verb Tense

	Past	Past Perfect	Present	Present Perfect	Future	Future Perfect
Time	started and completed in past	started and completed in past before some other past action	now	action started in past, continuing in present	will happen in future	will be completed in future
Form	regular verbs* add "d" or "ed" to base form	*had* + past participle	base form (third person singular adds "s")	*have* or *has* + past participle	*shall* or *will* + base form	*shall* or *will* + *have* + past participle
Examples	I ordered you ordered he/she/it ordered we ordered you ordered they ordered	I had ordered you had ordered he/she/it had ordered we had ordered you had ordered they had ordered	I order you order he/she/it orders we order you order they order	I have ordered you have ordered he/she/it has ordered we have ordered you have ordered they have ordered	I shall order you will order he/she/it will order we shall order you will order they will order	I shall have ordered you will have ordered he/she/it will have ordered we shall have ordered you will have ordered they will have ordered

*****Note:** For irregular verbs, consult your dictionary for past and past participle verb forms.

15.5   Adverbs

Just as adjectives modify nouns, *adverbs* modify verbs. Adverbs can also modify adjectives or other adverbs. Adverbs answer the questions "when," "how," "where," and "how much." Many adverbs end in *ly,* making them easy to identify.

When

Eric *now* knows the entire patient history.
Your prescription will be ready *soon.*

How

Lift the patient *slowly* onto the stretcher.
She *carefully* sterilized the instruments.

Where

The essential lab work will be completed *there.*
We found it here in the operating room.

How much

They complained *repeatedly* about the visiting hours.

15.6   Prepositions

Prepositions show the relationships between nouns or pronouns and other words in the sentence. This function is usually carried out by means of a *prepositional phrase,* which consists of a preposition and its object. Prepositional phrases almost always act as adverbs or adjectives.

The technician moved carefully *between* the hospital beds.

In this example, the preposition *between* shows the relationship between *moved,* the verb, and *beds. Beds* is the object of the preposition, and the entire phrase (*between the hospital beds*) acts as an adverb, telling where the technician moved. When pronouns are used as the object of a preposition, they must be in the objective case (see 15.2).

Yolanda placed a call *to her doctor.*
Greg searched high and low *for the medical records.*
Please write the prescription *for me.*

Frequently Used Prepositions

about	by	over
above	down	past
across	during	round
after	except	since
against	for	through
among	from	to
around	in	under
at	into	until
before	like	up
behind	of	upon
below	off	with
beside	on	within
between		without

15.7 Conjunctions

Conjunctions are words used to connect two words, phrases, or clauses. *Coordinating conjunctions* connect words, phrases, or clauses that are alike. Common examples are *and, but, for, or, nor,* and *yet.*

Dr. Lena Grant *and* Dr. Castell Bryant were honored at the banquet.
The medical secretaries like their jobs, *but* they want to continue their education.

Correlative conjunctions are pairs of words that connect two like words, phrases, or clauses. Common forms are *either/or, neither/nor, both/and, not/but, whether/or,* and *not only/but also.*

Either Dr. Vincent *or* her assistant will perform the routine surgery in the morning.
Neither Lourdes *nor* I remembered the appointment yesterday.

15.8 Problem Parts of Speech

Words sometimes sound alike but are used differently. Some words that serve both as adverbs and adjectives are often confused, and some nouns are confused with similar-sounding adjectives and adverbs. Use the following guide to avoid problems with these similar words.

Adapt/Adept/Adopt: The urology department will *adapt* this form to fit the purchasing department's new requirements. (adjust)

Mary and Leonard were both very *adept* at learning medical terminology. (skilled)

Karen and Craig McMeekin will *adopt* a son. (choose)

Allowed/Aloud:	Children may not be *allowed* to enter the obstetrics area. (permitted)
	Pam read the medical history *aloud* to her students. (out loud)
All Ready/ Already:	The mother and baby are *all ready* to go home now. (completely prepared)
	Have they left the hospital *already?* (before an understood time)
All Right/ Alright:	We were relieved to hear that they were *all right*. (satisfactory)
	Alright is not acceptable in standard English—do not use it. (HINT: Just as there is no word "alwrong," there is no word "alright.")
Among/ Between:	They always enjoy being *among* famous physicians. (*Among* is used when three or more persons or things are involved and no close relationship is indicated.)
	The choice is *between* Bart and Ricardo for Chief of Staff. (*Between* is used when two persons or things are involved; or with terms such as treaty, agreement, or discussion.)
Any One/ Anyone:	*Any one* of these courses will satisfy the requirements. (one of a set of persons or things)
	Has *anyone* seen the lab reports? (anybody)
Bad/Badly:	It looks *bad* for our Medicaid reports to be late. (After look, smell, and sound, *bad* is preferred.)
	This accident victim is *badly* in need of help. (very much)
Beside/Besides:	He stood *beside* me during the baby's birth. (next to)
	Besides my television, the thieves took the stereo and my medical bag. (in addition to)
Capital/Capitol:	The *capital* of Colorado is Denver. (*Capital* is used to mean a seat of government; a term in finance, accounting, and architecture; chief and first rate; capital letter; and capital punishment.)
	The signing of the new medical bill will take place in the *Capitol* Building at noon. (*Capitol* is used to mean the buildings used by Congress and State legislatures.)

Every One/ Everyone:	*Every one* of them had a full physical. (each one)
	Will *everyone* be coming to the hospital? (everybody)
Farther/ Further:	Your doctor's office is *farther* than I thought. (physical distance)
	His statement could not be *further* from the truth. (additional; greater distance in time or quantity)
Fewer/Less:	We had *fewer* debts in those days. (We had 10 debts then; we have 18 now.)
	We had *less* debt in those days. (We owed $2,100 then; we owe $4,800 now.)
Foreword/ Forward:	In the *foreword* of the book, the author mentions her years of medical research. (preface)
	Come *forward* a little into the light so I can see your new uniform. (toward the front, progressive)
Formally/ Formerly:	He was *formally* accepted as a member of the Medical Board after initiation. (in a formal manner)
	She was *formerly* the consulting physician. (previously, before)
Forth/Fourth:	From that day *forth,* she was never the same. (forward, onward in time)
	It was the *fourth* time I tried to contact the Urology Department. (after third)
Good/Well:	The chili smells *good*. (adjective only)
	Ann is *well* enough to join Karen at the game. (adjective or adverb)
Knew/New:	She *knew* Dr. Schaeffer before taking her class. (acquainted with)
	We filled our wing of the Medical Center with *new* furniture. (fresh, unused)
Last/Latest:	This is the *latest* announcement on AIDS. (most recent)
	Carmen McCrink was the *last* one to arrive for the Medical Council meeting. (final)
Later/Latter:	Enjoy yourself, it's *later* than you think. (After the usual or proper time.)
	Karen Paiva and J. Terrence Kelly were the two contestants; the *latter* was the winner. (second of two)

Leased/Least:	Maxine *leased* a condominium near the Omni Hospital. (rented)
	Arriving on time was the *least* of our worries today. (smallest)
Liable/Libel:	The hospital is *liable* for the patient's care. (responsible)
	The author was sued for *libel* after the book was published. (injury through written or printed statements)
Loose/Lose:	The connection was *loose,* and the EKG results were affected. (not secure)
	The surgical team did not want to *lose* a minute during the delicate surgery. (suffer a loss)
May Be/Maybe:	Your symptoms *may be* gone in the morning. (verb)
	Maybe we should call if the X rays don't arrive soon. (possibly—adverb)
Passed/Past:	To my surprise, I *passed* the medical terminology test. (proceeded beyond)
	In *past* treatment, the patient responded more quickly. (earlier time)
Personal/ Personnel:	My decision to leave the practice was a *personal* one. (private)
	The *personnel* at your laboratory seem very enthusiastic. (the employees)
Principal/ Principle:	Vera Worthington was the very popular *principal* of the school. (chief official, capital sum of money)
	It wasn't the decision that was made, rather it was the *principle* of the matter that was important to Dr. Joyce. (basic truth)
Real/Really:	Sarah Turbett was a *real* friend. (true, actual)
	Are you *really* going to support Medicare reform? (actually)
Some/Sum:	*Some* of the audience began to leave the gynecology lecture. (part)
	What is the *sum* of all your medical expenses? (total)
Some Time/ Sometime/ Sometimes:	It was *some time* before the nurse returned from intensive care. (a period of time)
	Sometime later this week, we will schedule a Glucose Tolerance Test. (at an unspecified time)

	Sometimes it is hard to understand written medical reports. (now and then)
Sure/Surely:	I am *sure* you can learn these medical abbreviations. (certain)
	Surely you don't want to quit now? (certainly)
Than/Then:	My blood pressure is higher now *than* it was when I first started to work. (as compared to)
	Wait until the ambulance stops; *then* you can get out safely. (at that time)
Their/There:	*Their* interest was in the patient's mental health. (pronoun)
	Write it *there* on the patient's chart. (in that place)
To/Too/Two:	Come *to* the hospital with me. (preposition)
	Ricky wants to come, *too*. (also)
	Two nurses were assigned to the same patient. (number following one)
Weak/Week:	He was too *weak* to climb any further. (not strong)
	This *week* we have a vacation from nursing school to celebrate the Fourth of July. (seven successive days)
Weather/ Whether:	The *weather* remained sunny during our entire medical conference. (state of the atmosphere)
	Whether or not we vote, our issue still cannot win. (regardless)

16

Eliminating Bias in Writing

All individuals are entitled to written materials which present members of both sexes, different ethnic groups, and all races with equal respect, dignity, and balance. To accomplish this, all written material should emphasize the potential of each individual and group. Today's writers are making an effort to eliminate many of the biases in writing that were common in the past. As you become aware of discriminatory practices in writing, you will find that there are many ways to avoid such bias.

16.1 Sexual Identifiers in Compound Nouns

Compound nouns very often contain the words *man* or *men* and have been used traditionally to refer to men and women alike. Such use is now considered discriminatory when applied to women. The U.S. Department of Labor helped to lead the way in the use of unbiased language in their 1975 publication, *Job Title Revisions to Eliminate Sex- and Age- Referent Language from the Dictionary of Occupational Titles.* The latest issues of the *Dictionary of Occupational Titles (DOT)* have been revised to eliminate all sexual identifiers.

Some alternatives for traditionally used compound nouns are listed below. For additional assistance, consult the *DOT.*

Avoid	**Use**
man, men, mankind	people, person(s), individual(s), human being(s), human race, humanity, women and men, human(s)
businessman(men)	business executive(s), business person(s), manager(s), merchant(s)
Congressman(men)	Congressional representative(s), member(s) of Congress
chairman(men)	chairperson(s), chair(s), department head(s), moderator(s), group leader(s)

salesmen	sales agents, salespeople, salespersons, sales representatives, sales force
workmen	workers
postman, mailman	postal clerk, mail carrier
repairman	repairer
foreman	supervisor
spokesman	spokesperson
maid	houseworker

In addition, substitute the following words which unnecessarily identify gender:

Avoid	Use
housewife	homemaker
poetess	poet
usherette	usher
co-ed	student
sculptress	sculptor
lady doctor or female doctor	doctor
male nurse	nurse

16.2 Sexual Identifiers in Generic Pronouns

The generic pronouns *he, his,* or *him* have often been used to indicate any member of a group, male or female. This practice is now avoided by many who think that it is unfair to use *he, his,* or *him* when discussing a group that is not all male. (Note: When the pronouns *they* or *their* are used, the sex of group members is not indicated.) One of the ways to avoid this bias is to eliminate the pronoun.

Avoid: Each doctor is responsible for his lab coat.

Use: Each doctor is responsible for personal lab coats.

Change from singular to plural.

Use: All doctors are responsible for their own lab coats.

Use words which do not indicate gender (you, one, person, individual, all).

Avoid: She must decide on a medical speciality.

Use: Each person must decide on a medical speciality.

Use job titles instead of the pronoun.

Avoid: She should be able to take vital statistics effectively.

Use: The nurse should be able to take vital statistics effectively.

Change the pronoun to an article.

Avoid: The doctor uses his patient charts to summarize his treatment decisions.

Use: The doctor uses patient charts to summarize the treatment decisions.

Add names to eliminate generic usage.

Avoid: The operating room nurse announced her engagement.

Use: The operating room nurse, Georgianna Stringer, announced her engagement.

Change from active to passive voice.

Avoid: She should inform the doctor immediately of any medical emergency.

Use: The doctor should be informed immediately of any medical emergency.

Repeat the noun instead of using the pronoun.

Avoid: If the patient has a question concerning the appointment, she can check with the medical receptionist.

Use: If the patient has a question concerning the appointment, the patient can check with the medical receptionist.

If the methods mentioned above fail, use both pronouns. Do this as a last resort, since including both the male and female pronouns is awkward.

Avoid: A medical student's goal is to complete his medical training.

Use: A medical student's goal is to complete his or her medical training.

16.3 Sexual Identifiers in Bibliographies

A recent trend is to eliminate sexual identifiers in published bibliographies by using author initials instead of first names.

Lamb, M. M. *Word Studies.* Cincinnati, OH: South-Western Publishing Co., 1971.

16.4 Age Identifiers

The latest *DOT* edition also eliminates implied age bias in occupational titles:

Avoid	Use
stock boy	stock clerk
bus boy	dining room attendant
curb girl	curb attendant

REFERENCES

U. S. Department of Labor. *Job Title Revisions to Eliminate Sex- and Age-Referent Language from the Dictionary of Occupational Titles,* 3d ed. Washington: U. S. Government Printing Office, 1975.

17

Punctuation

Punctuation helps the writer to show the reader such things as where to pause, what to emphasize, and what is possessive. Used correctly, punctuation adds to the meaning of written material.

The most commonly used punctuation marks are the apostrophe, colon, comma, hyphen, parentheses, period, quotation marks, and semicolon. The less commonly used punctuation marks include the ampersand, asterisk, brace or brackets, dash, diagonal or slash, exclamation mark, question mark, and underscore or italics.

17.1 Ampersand

The ampersand is used primarily with forms or tables. While not generally used in business correspondence, an exception is made when the ampersand is part of the official name of an organization.

Kaufman & Roberts   Eisenberg & Rojas

17.2 Apostrophe

The apostrophe is used to indicate possession and to show where letters were eliminated in contractions. Apostrophes also symbolize feet and minutes in measurements, and are used to form the plurals of letters, abbreviations, and symbols.

Possession. For singular and plural nouns not ending in *s*, add *'s*.

Kathie's horse   Nicky's car
children's program   women's vote

237

For singular nouns ending in *s*, add *'s*

Lourdes's address   Mercedes's new car
the hostess's uniform

Note: Some people prefer to use *'s* only when the singular noun ending in *s* is one syllable:

my boss's apartment house   the dress's zipper

For more than one syllable, or when the following word begins with the *s* or *z* sound, another option is to use the apostrophe alone:

Mercedes' new car   Lourdes' address
Tom Adams' superstitions

For plural nouns ending in *s*, add only the apostrophe:

contestants' prizes (prizes of the contestants)
boys' coats (coats of the boys)
golfers' behavior (behavior of the golfers)

For indefinite pronouns, add *'s:*

someone's shoes   anybody's license

For word groups, add *'s* to the last word of the group:

mother-in-law's gift   anyone else's advice
Secretary of Education's proposal

For joint ownership add *'s* to the last name:

Alan and Joan's house
(The house that Alan and Joan both own.)

For separate ownership, add *'s* to each name:

Alan's and Joan's cars.
(The cars that Alan and Joan each own.)

Some organization names do not use the apostrophe. Always follow the examples used in the organization's correspondence or letterhead.

United States Postal Service
Dade County Federal School Employees Credit Union

Contractions. Apostrophes are used to indicate missing letters or figures in contractions.

don't (do not)   haven't (have not)
won't (would not)   isn't (is not)
he'll (he will)   Class of '88 (1988)

Note: Do not confuse contractions with possessive pronouns. Possessive pronouns do not use the apostrophe.

Possessive Pronoun   **Contraction**

their   they're (they are)
its   it's (it is)
whose   who's (who is)

Feet and Minutes. Apostrophes are used to indicate feet and minutes.

16 feet, 5 inches 16'5"
8 minutes, 3 seconds 8'3"

Plurals. Apostrophes are used to indicate the plurals of letters, abbreviations, or symbols.

A's   CPA's   5's   #'s   ABC's

17.3 Asterisk

The *asterisk* is used to signal the inclusion of a footnote pertaining to an item within the written text. The asterisk is repeated before the actual footnote at the bottom of the same page. Second or third footnotes can be indicated with two or three asterisks.

Chuck Klingensmith
Richard Spivak*
Rene Gilbert
Eurie Davis
Nellie Quincy**
Harry Hoffman
Ray Pick
(At the bottom of the same page:)
*Class of '64
**Presidential Scholarship

Use three asterisks (typed with no spaces) to indicate an unprintable word.

The athlete's sentiments, "You ***," were carried on national television.

Use three asterisks (typed with spaces in between) to indicate the omission of an entire paragraph within quoted material.

The medical team was pleased to note the definite downward trend in the levels of cholesterol before the end of the research period.
* * *
In the end, the research team concluded that the drug was very effective in treating heart disease.

Note that an entire paragraph has been omitted between the end of the first paragraph and the beginning of the third.

17.4 Brace/Brackets

Use the brace (two or more parentheses) to indicate headings in legal documents.

The State of Michigan   ]
        vs   ]   as to
Albert Schlazer   ]

Use brackets to show information included for clarification.

The surgeon used the Lempert perforator [the latest model] during the flawless surgical procedure.

Use brackets with the word *sic* to show that a surprising word or error was quoted intentionally.

The newspaper headlines proclaimed, "Higher Costs Expected in New Medicle [sic] Treatment."

Use brackets to indicate insertions provided by someone other than the writer.

The Houston Medical Center [founded in 1812] is adding a new wing to its southernmost building.

Use brackets to indicate parenthetical expressions contained within parenthetical expressions.

The doctor requested that the next time he goes to Atlanta (Pediatric Surgeons Conference, April 19 and 20 [keynote speaker]), I make reservations at a different hotel.

17.5 Colon

Use the colon to separate an introductory phrase from illustration(s) that follow.

Family members included the following: Craig McMeekin, Karen McMeekin, Scotty McMeekin, and Holly Pam McMeekin.
Her favorite foods are high in carbohydrates: ice cream, bananas, candy, and bread.
The DPT immunization includes vaccine for the following:
Diphtheria
Pertussis
Tetanus

Note that the illustrations repeat or identify the introductory phrase. The introductory phrase often begins with *as follows, such as,* or *as listed*. The introductory phrase should not end with a preposition or a verb.

Within a sentence, there is no space before a colon and two spaces following. The colon is also used to introduce a complete sentence quotation:

The patient said: "The chemotherapy treatments make me nauseous."

The colon is used in expressions of time, biblical references, and ratios.

3:00 p.m.   John 3:16   a ratio of 3:1

The colon is used following the salutation of a business letter using mixed punctuation.

Dear Dr. Porter:

17.6 Comma

One of the most frequently used punctuation marks is the comma. The comma indicates a pause within a sentence and clarifies meaning.

As the effect of the drug hit, Mary Beth passed out.
As the effect of the drug hit Mary, Beth passed out.

The week before the Super Bowl, sales were low.
The week before, the Super Bowl sales were low.

While the correct use of the comma can improve writing, be cautious: overuse or incorrect use can confuse the reader.

Use the comma to set off an introductory word, phrase, or clause at the beginning of a sentence (optional).

Therefore, the time to act is now.
When an emergency exists, remain calm.
But: Remain calm when an emergency exists.

In spite of her broken leg, Ruth Greenfield attended.
But: Ruth Greenfield attended in spite of her broken leg.

For a young child, staying in the hospital can be a frightening experience.
But: Staying in the hospital can be a frightening experience for a young child.

Nonetheless, the nurses accepted the compromise.

Yes, the X rays show the femur is fractured.

Use commas to set off words or phrases that are in apposition to (repeat or identify) the preceding noun or noun phrase.

Dr. M. Glenn Tripplett, chief of staff, arrived early.
The nearest hospital, Harvey General, was five miles away.
Medical Center Campus honored Dr. George Hedgespeth, their dean of administration.

Use a comma to separate the two main clauses of a compound sentence. Each clause should have its own subject. Coordinating conjunctions such as *and, but, for, nor, or, so,* and *yet* are used to join the two clauses.

The patient had symptoms indicating bronchitis, and the doctor strongly advised against continued smoking.
He did not agree that he should lose weight, nor would he participate in the rest of his treatment program.
The prognosis was not good, but the patient responded beautifully following surgery.

When one of the main clauses has additional punctuation, most good writers prefer to use a semicolon to separate the two clauses. However, a comma may still be acceptable.

Prior to the opening of the football season, the doctor tested all of the athletes; but the examinations revealed none of the serious knee problems that had been anticipated.

Use commas to separate words, phrases, and clauses in a series.

The doctor requested the DeBakey clamp, forceps, needle holder, scissors, and tunneler.

The pregnant patient began labor, fed her family, packed a suitcase, and arrived at the hospital just in time for the birth of her baby.

The new gowns for Pediatrics were red, blue, green and white, orange, and yellow.

While the final comma in a series (preceding the final *and*) is considered optional, many prefer to use it for clarity. Notice what happens to the last example when the final comma is omitted:

The new gowns for Pediatrics were red, blue, green and white, orange and yellow.

Are there orange and yellow gowns, or gowns of orange and gowns of yellow? Always use the comma in such instances to avoid confusion.

Use a comma when introducing a quotation.

The patient called to ask, "Are my test results in yet?"

Use commas to set off words, clauses, or phrases within a sentence.

It was determined, however, that further treatment was unnecessary.

The nursing home personnel, not the patients, identified the areas needing attention.

It is the only way, I believe, to submit the claim.

Use commas to separate two or more adjectives modifying the same noun if you can insert *and* between them.

The technician handled the emergency in a calm, efficient manner. (calm and efficient)

It was her favorite old straw hat. (not old and straw hat)

Commas are used in numbers for clarity.

5,839,500   1,244 $99,439.88

Use commas to set off dates and to separate city and state names.

Monday, August 18, 19—
Los Angeles, California

January 15, 19—
Portland, Maine

Use commas to set off titles and degrees from personal names and to separate the abbreviations *Inc.* and *Ltd.* from company names.

Zelda Rosenwald, D.O., introduced the speaker.

Bullotta & Bryant, Inc.   Wiggins, Ltd.
Oscar Addison, Jr.   Janet Seitlin, J.D.

Note: A new trend makes such commas optional. Follow the preferences expressed by organizations and individuals.

17.7 Dash

Use the dash to indicate an abrupt pause or an interruption in thought.

I want you to know that the next time—but then, time is short.
The size of the incision—less than 1/2 inch—was a surprise to the patient.

Use the dash to emphasize a parenthetical expression.

It was October 12—the longest day in my life—when I finally received my test results.

Use the dash before the author's name which follows a quotation.

To be or not to be: that is the question.
—Shakespeare

17.8 Slash

Use the slash to indicate a choice or option between two words.

For her birthday celebration, the doctor requested filet mignon and/or lobster.

This usage should be avoided in formal writing.

Use the slash with numbers.

date (informal):   4/19/55
fractions: 1/4
time periods: 78/79

Use the slash with abbreviations.

in care of: c/o
with: w/
without: w/o

17.9 Exclamation Mark

Use the exclamation mark to indicate strong feelings or to issue a command.

Please help me! I have to know!
Come here! Now!
Code Blue!

Use the exclamation mark following interjections.

Wow!	Terrific!	Sure!

17.10 Hyphen

Hyphenation is discussed in Chapter 19. See the following list:

Word Division—see 19.1, p. 260.
Compound Adjectives—see 19.2, p. 261.
Compound Nouns—see 19.3, p. 261.
Numbers—see 19.4, p. 262.
Ranges—see 19.5, p. 262.
Suspended Hyphenation—see 19.6, p. 262.
Family Relationships—see 19.7, p. 262.
Other Uses—see 19.8, p. 262.

17.11 Parentheses

Parentheses are used to enclose nonessential or illustrative material. They are always used in pairs.

The meeting (I thought it would go on forever) lasted until 9:00 p.m.
The patient was delighted with the results of the new treatment (which was only discovered six months ago).
Henry Ford Hospital (founded in 1885) is known for cardiac research.

Note that the elimination of the information in the parentheses does not change the meaning of the sentence.

Use parentheses to set off numbers or letters that indicate divisions within a sentence.

To place the call (a) dial the local access number, (b) dial the area code and telephone number of your party, and (c) input the authorization code following the tone.

Use parentheses in outlines to set off the letters and numbers that mark subdivisions of lesser importance.

I. Education
  A. Medical Education
    1. Medical Office Employee Training
      a. Medical Communications
        (1) Medical Correspondence
          (a) Letter Formats

Use parentheses to enclose figures added to clarify written-out numbers.

The inventory indicated that thirty-four (34) sheets, sixty-seven (67) pillow cases, and eighty-eight (88) towels were destroyed in the fire.
The quoted salary was eighty-five thousand dollars ($85,000) per year.

Use parentheses to enclose abbreviations following written-out names.

The doctor is a member of both the American Medical Association (AMA) and the Spanish American League Against Discrimination (SALAD).

Use parentheses to enclose punctuation added within a sentence for emphasis or irony.

He reported that his highly prized (!) manuscript was missing.

Parentheses may also be used in place of commas or dashes to give the set-off material less emphasis. Note that punctuation which is part of the material included within parentheses is included inside the parentheses, while punctuation which is part of the sentence as a whole is placed outside the parentheses.

The patient was delighted with the results of the new treatment (which had been discovered only six months earlier).

17.12 Period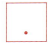

Use the period at the end of complete sentences.

Dr. Suzanne Richter performed surgery on Trine Englebretzen, the liver transplant recipient who stole the hearts of Miami.
The cold and flu season increased the need to work patients into an already crowded appointment schedule.

Use the period at the end of sentences where understood words have been eliminated.

Come here, please.
Sit here.
Sure.

Use the period at the end of indirect questions.

The patients asked when lunch would be served.
I wonder when the group from Jamaica will arrive.

Use the period with some initials and abbreviations.

Mrs.	M. Duane Hansen
Robert H. McCabe	D. E. Miot
Ms.	Inc.

The use of periods with abbreviations varies. The following abbreviations, for example, should be written without periods:

YMCA   NATO   CPA

Many of these abbreviations are *acronyms,* words made from the initials of names. Acronyms are usually written in all capital letters without periods.

National Organization for Women	NOW
Skill Training Improvement Program	STIP

As you have seen, abbreviations are sometimes written with periods and sometimes written without periods. Sometimes they are written in all lowercase letters, sometimes in all capitals, and sometimes as a combination of both. Sometimes, more than one way of writing abbreviations is acceptable.

M.D.	MD	D.O.	DO
Ph.D.	c.o.d.	COD	a.m.

The keys to the correct use of periods with abbreviations are to (a) always follow the preferences expressed by the named individual or group, (b) always be consistent in the use of each abbreviation, and (c) always consult your dictionary when you need assistance.

The American Medical Association and the American Osteopathic Association prefer that no periods be used with medical abbreviations.

APF   Ca   EKG   FBS   HCG   kg   lab   MA

Use periods with the letters and numbers that mark outline segments, except for those enclosed in parentheses.

I. Ethics
   A. Medical Ethics
      1. Patient Rights
         a. Confidentiality
            (1) Releasing Patient Information
                (a) Releasing Information to Insurance Providers

Use periods following letters or numbers that mark listed items. Space twice after these periods. The period at the end of the listed item itself, however, is optional. Be consistent.

Anabel's complaints included three symptoms:
1. Headache
2. Insomnia
3. Loss of appetite

Dr. Marcia Captan told the Medical Technology graduates that their success following graduation depended upon three things:
A. Continued education.
B. Eagerness to learn on the job.
C. Hard work.

Use three periods, an *ellipsis,* to indicate an omission in quoted material. Use four periods to indicate omission at the end of a sentence.

The televised report stated: "The fire was discovered early . . . ambulances have been dispatched to the scene . . . firefighters do not yet know what caused the blaze."
"The symptoms were painful . . . ."

Note: Periods are always written within quotation marks.

Use periods with dollars and cents, percentages, and decimals.

4.5%   .0068   1,766.883 $13.82 $1.98   *But:* $500

Do not use periods with roman numerals within text, nicknames, or radio and television station call letters.

VII   Ed   Sam   WTVS   NBC

Chapter 17—Punctuation   **249**

17.13   Question Mark   ?

Use the question mark following a direct question.

Where is the doctor? Are you all right?
The patient asked the doctor, "Will I have to go to the hospital?"

Use the question mark to express doubt.

This is the happiest (?) day of my life.

Use the question mark for a series of questions with the same subject and verb.

Is the equipment working? correctly? efficiently?

17.14   Quotation Marks   " "

Use quotation marks in pairs to indicate direct quotations of spoken or written material. Quotation marks indicate exact duplication of the material in quotes.

"History was made," reported Dr. DeVries, "when Dr. Barney Clark pioneered the artificial heart."
"The entire family supported Dr. Clark's decision to try the artificial heart," Mrs. Una Loy Clark told the students.
After hearing Mrs. Clark's speech, the student said, "This is truly a story of family strength, love, and courage."

Note: The placement of punctuation and quotation marks depends on where the quotation comes within the sentence.

Use quotation marks in pairs to indicate the definition of a word or phrase from another language.

It was a real faux pas—"a tactless remark!"

Use quotation marks in pairs to indicate the titles of articles, speeches, parts of books or periodicals, short poems, and radio and television shows.

"The Creative Side of Word Processing" led off the January issue of *PC World*.
Following the increased interest in trivia games, "Jeopardy" benefited from larger audiences.

In typewritten material, when a quotation is more than four or five lines, it is identified as a quotation by indenting five spaces from each margin. In such instances, quotation marks are not used—the indentions take the place of the punctuation.

Use the apostrophe as a single quotation mark to indicate a quotation within a quotation.

The patient reported, "The prescription label reads, 'Take one tablet every three hours.' "

17.15 Semicolon

Use the semicolon to separate independent clauses within the same (compound) sentence when the clauses are not joined by a conjunction.

The insurance representative will be here this afternoon; there is a new form we must use for claims.
All office personnel should be here by 8:00 a.m.; the doctor wants the office closed at 3:30 p.m.

Use the semicolon to separate independent clauses joined by a conjunction when either clause has internal punctuation.

Following the examination, the doctor spoke privately with the patient; but the next morning she wanted to see the doctor again.
Please come to the meeting at the health center; and, if you have a chance, invite Dr. Brookner.

Use the semicolon to separate independent clauses when the clauses are joined by a conjunctive adverb such as *however, therefore, still, accordingly,* or *nonetheless.*

During Paella '84 the ambulance stood by; fortunately, it was never needed.
The child dialed the emergency number; however, he was confused about his exact address.

Use the semicolon to separate listed items when any item contains an internal comma.

The doctor's enviable itinerary included stops in Miami, Florida; San Francisco, California; Honolulu, Hawaii; and Peking, China.

17.16 Underscore or Italics

Use the underscore or italics to emphasize a word or phrase.

Elsa finished *first* in the 10K run.
The doctor stressed the importance of warming up *before* the game.

Use the underscore or italics to indicate the titles of books, magazines, newspapers, plays, musical works, long poems, paintings, and movies.

The *Miami Herald* reported the results of the grand jury investigation.
I consulted the *Reference Manual for Office Personnel* and I found the answer that I needed.

18

Capitalization

Capitalization is the process of using capital (uppercase) letters for emphasis. Capitalized words demand more attention, and thus become more important within the context of the surrounding words.

18.1 Basics

ALWAYS capitalize the first word in a sentence. This indicates to the reader where a new sentence begins.

The doctor needs your assistance immediately!
Patients often need encouragement during their treatment.

ALWAYS capitalize the exact names of specific persons, places, or things.

Dr. Elizabeth Lundgren will deliver the lecture.
He had his surgery at Baptist Hospital.
Reyes Syndrome is a concern for parents with young children.

It is important to note that capitalization is sometimes used to emphasize certain words. However, over-capitalization will reduce the value of this important tool.

18.2 Business Letters

Within a medical business letter, the following capitalization rules always apply:

Date.   Capitalize the first letter of the month.

December 18, 19--

Inside Address.   Capitalize the first letter of the personal or professional titles preceding names; professional titles on a line by themselves; names of individuals; names of companies or organizations; names of streets, avenues, and cities; and both letters of the two-letter state abbreviation. (NOTE: When capitalizing several words in a title, do not capitalize articles (the, a, an), short prepositions (four or fewer letters), or short conjunctions (and, as, nor, or, but).

> Dr. Irene Canal-Petersen
> Director of Research
> The Upjohn Manufacturing Company
> 2834 Avenida del Sol
> Barceloneta, PR 00617-3482
>
> Dr. Lourdes Rabade
> Obstetrics and Gynecology
> Palmetto General Hospital
> 2001 W. 68 Street
> Hialeah, FL 33016-1234

Salutation. Capitalize the first word in a business letter salutation, as well as the title and last name.

> Dear Dr. Schram:
> Dear Ms. Kerr-Stewart
>
> Ladies and Gentlemen:

Headings. Capitalize the first letter in attention and subject lines. That is, capitalize *Attention* and *Subject* and the words that follow. (*Subject* may also be typed in all capitals.)

> Attention: Technician Byrne
>
> Subject: Laboratory Procedures
>
> SUBJECT: Johnson, Joseph

Within the Body of the Letter. Follow all other capitalization rules covered in this unit.

Complimentary Close. Capitalize only the first word in the complimentary close.

> Sincerely,
>
> Yours truly,
>
> Sincerely yours

18.3 Business Organizations and Institutions

Always follow the preference of an organization for the capitalization of its name. The official letterhead is a reliable guide.

Capitalize the specific names of associations, churches, clubs, colleges and universities (including divisions within a college or university), companies, conventions, fraternities and sororities, hospitals, independent committees and boards, institutions, libraries, schools, synagogues, and political parties.

Mt. Sinai Medical Center	Democratic National Committee
Coppolechia Medical Library	Temple Beth Or
Wayne County Medical Association	Michigan State University
	Department of Neurology
American Medical Association	McNeil Pharmaceutical
Variety Childrens Hospital	Psychology Department

18.4 Education

Capitalize the titles of specific courses, but do not capitalize references to general academic subject areas (except languages).

Specific Course: All students are required to take Medical Terminology I before graduation.
A new course, Advanced Sports Medicine, will be added.
General Subject Area: Nelson wants to take a course in pediatrics.
Utako is studying Spanish.

When used with the name of an individual, an academic degree is capitalized. When used with the word *degree,* however, academic degrees are not capitalized.

With Name: Victoria Sigler, Juris Doctor, is an excellent attorney.
With Degree: Most colleges offer both the bachelor of science and the bachelor of arts degrees.

18.5 Government

Government Bodies. Capitalize the names of countries and international organizations, as well as the national, state, county, city, and local bodies and agencies within them.

the United Nations	Germany
Ft. Collins School District	Department of Education
the Johnson Administration	the Utah Legislature
the Cabinet	

Capitalize the short forms of international and national bodies and their major divisions when the reference is clear.

the Court (United States Supreme Court)
the Agency (Central Intelligence Agency)
the House (House of Representatives)
the Department (Department of Education)
the Bureau (Federal Bureau of Investigation)

Officials and Titles. Titles of international, national, and state government officials are capitalized when they immediately precede a specific individual's name and are part of the name. (Ambassador, Attorney General, Chief Justice, Chief of Staff, Governor, King, Lieutenant Governor, President, Prime Minister, Prince, Princess, Queen, Secretary-General of the United Nations, Secretary of State, Vice-President) These titles are not capitalized, however, when used to refer to an entire class of officials.

State Senator Carrie Meek called me today about the HMO Bill.
President John F. Kennedy was responsible for starting the Peace Corps.
But: The candidates for treasurer must have budgetary experience.

A title used in place of a personal name is capitalized only for toasts or informal introductions.

Ladies and gentlemen, the President of the United States.

Titles following a personal name (or used alone instead of a name) are generally lowercased.

Sis Smith, administrative assistant, took charge.

Laws, treaties, bills, and acts which have been formally adopted are capitalized when used with their full title, but do not capitalize the shortened form used in place of the full name.

Full Title	**Short Form**
Public Law 88-6578	the law
the Panama Canal Treaty	the treaty
Senate Bill 9758	the bill

Note this exception:

The Constitution of the United States of America

18.6 Hyphenation

Capitalize hyphenated words in the same way you would capitalize those words if they stood alone.

It was mid-April before her condition began to improve.
The Spanish-speaking nurses are helping me learn Spanish.
It was David Harris's thirty-eighth annual Treasure Hunt.

At the beginning of a sentence, however, remember to capitalize the first letter of the hyphenated word.

Mothers-in-law take too much abuse.
Up-to-date equipment is a must for accurate diagnosis.

For hyphenated names, capitalize each word except articles (*the, a, an*), short prepositions (four or fewer letters), and short conjunctions (*and, as, but, nor, or*).

Miami-Dade Community College
Slow-and-Easy Rowing Machine
President-Elect Stokes
Over-the-Hill Gang
Come-with-Eastern Vacation Package

18.7 Nouns Including Letters and Numbers

Nouns followed by letters or numbers should be capitalized. The exceptions are *line, note, page, size*, and *verse*; these should be lowercase. Capitalizing the noun *paragraph* is optional.

Appendix C	line 17
Article VI	page 116
Bulletin 88	size 16
Chapter XVIII	note 3
Column 2	verse 6
Diagram 9	Exhibit D
Paragraph 9	paragraph 9
Figure 79	Invoice 33-959
Lesson 44	Room 1515

18.8 Persons

Names should be capitalized, spelled, and spaced exactly as the named individuals write them. A name containing a prefix such as *d', da, de, del, della, di, du, l', la, le, mac, mc, o', van,* or *von* can vary in capitalization and spacing. Follow the individual's preferences.

Zoila de Zayas	Patrick W. Gettings
Carol Ann Galsworthy	Ida Hernandez-Fumero
Peter J. Masiko, Jr.	Benjamin von Wooster

Titles of relatives are capitalized when they precede a name, or when they are used as a name. They are not capitalized, however, when they follow a possessive pronoun or when they simply describe a family relationship.

Please, Mother, come to my room.
My Uncle Ken works in the Pediatric Department.
Aunt Leota and Aunt Sammy visited me in the hospital.
But:
My cousin enrolled in a dietary technician program.
I have 16 aunts and uncles.

18.9 Personal and Professional Titles

Capitalize all formal titles when they precede a name.

Miss Barbara Ciamataro	Judge Margarita Esquiroz
Reverend Kenneth Long	President Robert McCabe

Do not capitalize such titles when they follow a name.

Robert McCabe, president	Beverly Creely, professor

Do not capitalize personal or professional titles when the name that follows is set off by commas (appositive).

The vice-president, Robert Hodges, will speak later.
But:
Vice-President Robert Hodges will speak later.

Do not capitalize occupational titles when they precede or follow personal names.

The introduction was made by surgeon Mark Edwards.
We had dinner at the home of Mercy Cobb, attorney.

When the occupational title is a specific job title, however, capitalize it.

Senior Editor John Adams is working with me on my book.

Generally, do not capitalize official titles when they follow a personal name or are used in place of a personal name. (Exceptions are made for high government titles—see Section 18.5.)

Annie Betancourt, president, will preside at the meeting.
Calling the group together was Richard Schinoff, dean.

Note: Some companies capitalize all or some of the titles of company officials. Always follow the procedures preferred by your employer, and respect the preferences of others regarding their own titles.

With the doctorate degree, use *Dr.* before the name or the academic abbreviation following the name.

Dr. William McNae   or   William McNae, D.O.
Incorrect: Dr. William McNae, D.O.

18.10 Places, Things, and Ideas

Capitalize the complete names of specific places, things, or ideas. (Do not capitalize articles, short prepositions, or short conjunctions used within these names unless they are the first word of the name.) Do not capitalize the short forms used in place of the full name.

Woodward Medical Center	the medical center
Jefferson Hospital	the hospital
Equal Rights Amendment	the amendment
Penobscot Building	the building
The Denver Post	the newspaper

18.11 Publications

Capitalize the principal words in titles of publications (books, magazines, journals, pamphlets, newspapers) and other artistic works (movies, plays, songs, paintings, sculptures, and poems). Titles of complete published works or complete artistic works (motion pictures, long musical compositions such as symphonies and concertos) are underscored, italicized, or typed in all capital letters.

Book: I find *Physicians' Desk Reference* a helpful aid.
I find the PHYSICIANS' DESK REFERENCE a helpful aid.
Magazine: Your first copy of *The Pediatrician* arrived.
Your first copy of THE PEDIATRICIAN arrived.
Newspaper: The *Newark Star Ledger* won the award.
The NEWARK STAR LEDGER won the award.
Symphony: We have tickets for tonight's performance of Beethoven's *Symphony No. 9 in D Minor.*
We have tickets for tonight's performance of Beethoven's SYMPHONY NO. 9 IN D MINOR.

The titles of songs, short poems, and television and radio programs are enclosed in quotation marks.

All of the patients watched "General Hospital" every afternoon.

18.12 Time

Capitalize the names of days and months.

Monday	December	Wednesday	June

Capitalize names of holidays or religious days.

Martin Luther King Day	Passover
Mother's Day	New Year's Eve

Capitalize the names of historical events and the nicknames of historical periods.

World War I   the Great Depression

Do not capitalize the names of decades and centuries unless they are part of a nickname.

the nineteen-sixties   the eighteenth century
 But: the Roaring Twenties

Do not capitalize seasons of the year unless they are part of a specific title or are personified.

spring fever   fall colors   summer sunshine
 But:
Spring and Summer Sale
Oh beautiful Spring, I enjoy your days.

19

Hyphenation

Hyphenation is the use of the hyphen (-) to provide clarity in the communications process.

19.1 Word Division

One of the most common uses of the hyphen is to divide long words at the end of a line so that all lines of a typewritten document are balanced. Before showing how such words are divided, however, it is important to review some DO NOTs of word division.

1. DO NOT divide unless necessary.

2. DO NOT divide one syllable words or very short words (5 or fewer letters) of more than one syllable. For example, do not divide the following words:

    help   item   would   title

3. DO NOT divide words if the divided words look strange or if the divided words would cause confusion for the reader.

4. DO NOT divide words if you leave only two letters on the first line, or if you carry only two letters to the next line.

5. DO NOT divide a word at the end of a page.

6. DO NOT divide words on consecutive lines or have many divided words on the same page. Remember that each divided word may cause a break in the reader's concentration or understanding.

With these cautions in mind, use the following guidelines for word division at the end of the typewritten line:

1. Divide words only between syllables. Consult your dictionary for syllable identification.

2. Divide at the syllable break that is as close as possible to the middle of the word. This makes the divided word easier to read, since half of the word will be on one line and half will be on the next line. (/ = syllable break)

Chapter 19—Hyphenation   **261**

in/ter/wo/ven   inter-woven
no/ta/tion/al   nota-tional
ir/re/spon/si/bil/i/ty   irrespon-sibility
la/ryn/go/cen/te/sis   laryngo-centesis
neu/ro/plas/ty   neuro-plasty
py/ro/phos/pha/tase   pyrophos-phatase

3. Divide at natural breaks to clarify meaning.

extracurricular   extra-curricular
introduction   intro-duction
bronchopulmonary   broncho-pulmonary
hemoglobinuria   hemo-globinuria
tracheoplasty   tracheo-plasty

4. If you must break a hyphenated word at the end of the line, divide at the hyphen.

mother-in-law   mother- in-law
jack-in-the-box   jack-in- the-box
Perma-hand silk suture   Perma- hand silk suture
DeBakey-Cooley retractor   DeBakey- Cooley retractor
Pels-Macht test   Pels- Macht test

19.2   Compound Adjectives

When two or more words work together as an adjective and precede the noun that they modify, use hyphens to join them.

first-rate performance
up-to-date results
top-of-the-line equipment

Since some compound adjectives are combined and written as one word, always consult your dictionary.

firsthand look
lowermost section

19.3   Compound Nouns

Like compound adjectives, compound nouns are written in several different ways. They may be written together, they may be written apart, or they may be hyphenated.

Together	**Apart**	**Hyphenated**
timecard	Ferris wheel	half-wit
livestock	sales receipt	know-it-all
flashlight	lead runner	president-elect

Consult your dictionary for assistance.

19.4 Numbers

When fractions are written out, use hyphens.

one-fourth
three-eighths

When numbers from 21 to 99 are written out, use hyphens.

twenty-one   forty-eight
ninety-nine

19.5 Ranges

Use hyphens to indicate ranges.

pages 16-18   1977-1985
March 12-31   Sections F-H

19.6 Suspended Hyphenation

When a series of hyphenated adjectives has a common base word and this word is shown only once, a suspended hyphen follows each adjective.

He missed his first-, second-, and third-period classes.

19.7 Family Relationships

With the prefix *great-* and the suffix *-in-law*, hyphenate the following family relationships:

great-grandmother
great-aunt
father-in-law
sister-in-law

However, with the prefixes *grand-*, *step-*, and *god-*, family relationships are written as one word.

grandfather
stepson
godmother

Half brother and *half sister* are written as two words.

19.8 Other Uses of the Hyphen

When *anti-* is followed by a word that is capitalized, a hyphen is used. Most other words formed with *anti-* are written as one word without hyphens.

anti-Semitic   anti-British
But: antiwar

It is common practice to hyphenate words formed with the prefixes *ex-* and *self-*.

ex-girlfriend   self-reliant

Words formed with the prefix *re-* are generally not hyphenated unless the meaning is unclear.

Re-cover the chair. (adds clarity)
But: She will recover.
re-creation of the mood (adds clarity)
But: recreation center
re-form the profile (adds clarity)
But: He promised to reform.

Appendix

COMMON MEDICAL TERMINOLOGY

For correct spelling and exact definition of a medical term, always consult a medical dictionary. Several are listed on pages 277-278. The following sections will provide you with some general definitions of common medical terminology.

Root Words or Combining Forms

A root word is the foundation of a medical term; it usually names a part of the body or substance. Combining forms accommodate the addition of another root word, a prefix, or a suffix to develop more precise medical terms.

abdomin	related to the abdomen abdominalgia—abdominal pain
adeno, aden	gland, glandular adenogenous—originating in glandular tissue
aer, aero	relating to air or gas aerated—charged with air
andro	male, masculine androgenous—giving birth to a boy
angio, angi	relating to blood or lymph vessels angiography—description of blood vessels
arterio, arteri	related to the artery arteriogram—X ray of the artery
bio	life biology—the study of life
brachy	short brachyodont—having short teeth

brady	slow bradycardia—slow heart beat
broncho, bronch, bronchi	air passages within the lungs bronchoplasty—surgical repair of any defect in the bronchi
caco, caci, cac	bad, ill cacogeusia—a bad taste
carcino, carcin	relating to cancer carcinoma—any type of cancer
cardio, cardi	relating to the heart cardiograph—an instrument for recording heart movement
cata	down cataphoria—a downward deviation of either eye while the other fixes
cephalo, cephal	relating to the head cephalopathy—any disease affecting the head or brain
chrom, chromat, chromato, chromo	color chromatoptometry—measurement of color perception
cyst, cysti, cysto	relating to the bladder or a cyst cystoma—a cystic tumor; a new growth containing cysts
cyto, cyt	cell cytology—the study of cells
dacryo, dacry	tears dacryorrhea—excessive flow of tears
dactylo, dactyl	fingers, sometimes toes dactyledema—swelling of the finger
dent, denti, dento	tooth denticle—a small tooth
derm, derma, dermat, dermato, dermo	relating to the skin dermatome—an instrument for cutting the skin

diplo	double, twin diplopia—double vision
ecto, ect	outer, on the outside ectopic—a pregnancy out of the cavity of the uterus
gastro, gastr	relating to the stomach gastrocele—hernia of the stomach
gluco	relating to glucose (sugar) glucocorticoids—cortical hormones that maintain blood sugar levels
glyco	relating to sugars in general glycosuria—sugar in the urine
gyno, gyn, gyne, gyneco	relating to woman, female gynecology—the branch of medicine relating to diseases of women
hem, hema, hemat, hemato	relating to blood hematocele—a blood cyst
hepat, hepatico, hepato	relating to the liver hepatocele—hernia of the liver
hetero, heter	other, different heterosexuality—attraction toward the opposite sex
homo	same, alike homosexuality—attraction toward the same sex
hydro, hydr	relating to water hydrocephalus—excessive fluid in the cerebral ventricles
hystero, hyster	womb, uterus hysterectomy—removal of the uterus
idio	private, peculiar to, separate, distinct idiomuscular—relating to the muscles alone, independent of the nervous control
kinesi, kinesio, kineso	motion photokinetic—relating to movement caused by light
latero	lateral, to one side laterodeviation—a bending to one side

leuko, leuk	white leukocyte—white blood cell
litho, lith	stone or calculus, calcification lithoid—resembling a calculus or stone
macro, macr	large, long macroglossia—enlargement of the tongue
mal	bad, ill malabsorption—imperfect or inadequate gastrointestinal absorption
mega, megal, megalo	large, oversize megacolon—enlarged or dilated colon
melan, melano	black or extreme darkness melanoma—malignant pigmented mole or tumor
meno	relating to menses menorrhea—normal menstruation
myo	muscle myocarditis—inflammation of the muscular walls of the heart
naso	relating to the nose nasosinusitis—inflammation of the nasal cavities
nephro, nephr	relating to the kidney nephremorrhagia—hemorrhage from or into the kidney
neuro	nerve or nervous system neurectomy—excision of a segment of a nerve
oculo	relating to the eye oculonasal—relating to the eyes and the nose
odyn, odyno	pain hysterodynia—pain in the uterus
odont, odonto	relating to teeth odontotomy—cutting into the crown of a tooth
oligo, olig	few, less, small, a little oliguria—scanty urination
opistho	backward, behind opisthotic—behind the ear
osteo, ost, oste	relating to the bone osteocyte—bone cell

path, patho, pathy	disease pathogen—any virus, microorganism, or other substance causing disease
phobia	fear ochlophobia—fear of crowds
pneum, pneuma, pneumat, pneumato	relating to air, lungs, breath pneumonia—inflammation of the lungs
psycho, psych	mind psychiatry—treatment of diseases of the mind
pyo	pus pyonephrosis—pus in the kidney
sarco	resemblance to flesh, muscular substance sarcocele—a fleshy tumor
sclero, scler	relating to the sclera (white of the eye) scleritis—inflammation of the sclera
spasm	involuntary muscle contraction enterospasm—intestinal muscle contraction
steno	narrowness, constriction stenostomia—narrowness of the oral cavity
toxico, tox, toxi, toxo	poison toxicology—the science of poisons
vas, vasculo, vaso	relating to a blood vessel vasopuncture—puncturing a vessel with a needle

Medical Prefixes

A prefix is one or more syllables at the beginning of a medical term that modifies the meaning of the term. Prefixes are used to indicate quantity, location, or direction.

a-, an-	not, without, less analgesia—the absence of the normal sense of pain
ab-	away from, off abduct—to move away from the axis of the body

ad-	toward, to increase adduct—bringing to or toward the median plane of the body
ambi-	round, both, all (both) sides ambilateral—relating to both sides
ana-	up, toward, apart anabiosis—resuscitation after apparent death
ante-	before, prior antepartum—before labor or childbirth
anti-, ant-	against, opposing, curative antiallergic—preventing an allergic reaction
auto-, aut-	self, same autism—morbid self-absorption
bi-, bis-	twice, double, two biped—two-footed
circum-	around, circular motion circumduction—movement of a part of the body in a circular direction
con-, com-, co-	together with concrescence—in dentistry, the union of the roots of a tooth, or of two adjacent teeth
contra-	against, counter, opposed contraception—the prevention of conception or impregnation
de-	from, not, down dehydrate—to lose water
di-	two, twice diphasic—occurring in two phases or stages
dia-	through, throughout, completely diadermic—through unbroken skin
dis-	negative, apart, absence of disorientation—loss of the sense of familiarity of one's surroundings
dys-	difficult, bad dyspnea—difficulty or distress in breathing
en-, em-	in, into, on embalm—to treat a dead body with balsams or antiseptics to preserve it from decay

endo-, ento-	within, inside, inner endocardia—the innermost layer of the heart
epi-	upon, following, in addition, over, on epiglottis—lidlike structure that covers the entrance to the larynx
ex-	out of, from, away from expectorate—to spit
exo-	exterior, external, outward exopathy—disease produced by some cause outside the body
extra-	without, outside of extracellular—outside of the cells
hemi-	one-half hemiparesis—slight paralysis affecting one side only
hyper-	increased, above normal, extreme, excessive hypertension—high blood pressure
hypo-, hyp-	under, decreased, below normal hypotension—low blood pressure
in-, im-	not, in, within, inside infertility—diminished or absent fertility; relative sterility
infra-	implies below infrapatellar—below the patella (kneecap)
inter-	between, among interdigital—between the fingers or toes
intra-	within intrahepatic—within the liver
intro-	in, into introgastric—leading or passed into the stomach
meso-, mes-	middle mesencephalon—the midbrain
meta-	after, between, over metacarpals—bones of the hand between the fingers and the wrist
micro-	small microcolon—small colon
mono-, mon-	one, single monocyte—a large leuckocyte with one nucleus

multi-	many, much multicellular—composed of many cells
neo-	new, recent neonate—newborn
ortho-	normal, straight, right orthodontics—branch of dentistry concerned with the straightening of teeth
pan-	all, entire, every panophobia—fear of everything
para-	beside, along side of paracystic—alongside or near the bladder
per-	through percutaneous—through unbroken skin
peri-	around, about peribronchial—surrounding a bronchus
poly-	much, many polyarthritis—simultaneous inflammation of several joints
post-	after, behind postpartum—after childbirth or delivery
pre-	before premorbid—preceding the occurrence of disease
pro-	before, in front of procephalic—the front of the head
proto-	first in a series, highest in rank protospasm—a spasm beginning in one limb and gradually becoming more general
pseudo-, pseud-	deceptive resemblance, false pseudomnesia—an impression of memory for an event that did not occur
re-	again, backward reaction—response to stimuli
retro-	backward, behind retroflexed—bent backward
semi-	one-half seminormal—one-half of the normal
sub-	beneath, under, below, less than normal subcutaneous—beneath the skin

super- above, excessive
superolateral—at the side and above

supra- above
supraintestinal—above the intestine

syn-, sym- with, together, joined, union
syndrome—a group of signs and symptoms that collectively characterize a particular disease or abnormal condition

trans- across, through
transection—cutting across

tri- three
tricellular—having three cells

uni- one, single, not paired
unilobar—having one lobe

Medical Suffixes

A suffix is one or more syllables at the end of a medical term that clarifies or alters the meaning of that word. Suffixes also indicate the part of speech: noun, verb, or adjective.

-algia relating to pain, painful condition
neuralgia—severe pain along the course of a nerve

-ase enzyme
oxidase—one of a group of enzymes in animal and vegetable tissues that bring about oxidation

-cele swelling, hernia
cystocele—hernia of the bladder

-cyte cell
macrocyte—a large cell

-ectomy removal of any organ or gland from the body
tonsillectomy—removal of the entire tonsil

-emia blood
anemia—a blood disorder with less than normal red blood cells

-fuge to drive away, flight
centrifuge—an apparatus which separates solid particles in a fluid

-genesis origin, production
chondrogenesis—the formation of cartilage

-gram	picture, tracing, mark, recording neurogram—imprint on the brain left behind after every mental activity
-graph	an instrument to record, trace micrograph—an instrument that magnifies microscopic movements of a diaphragm
-ia, -iasis, -osis	abnormal or diseased condition or state lithiasis—condition marked by the formation of stones
-itis	inflammation of appendicitis—inflammation of the appendix
-logia, -logy	science of, study pharmacology—science of drug sources, appearances, chemistry, actions, and uses
-lysis	setting free, disintegration, dissolution hemolysis—the alteration or destruction of red blood cells
-oid	to form a like shape, resembling myoid—resembling muscle
-oma	tumor carcinoma—cancerous tumor
-osis	condition, process or state, usually abnormal or diseased dermatosis—any skin disorder
-plasia	formation, growth hyperplasia—excessive increase in tissue growth
-plegia	paralysis cardioplegia—paralysis of the heart
-rrhagia	excessive or unusual discharge menorrhagia—abnormal bleeding during menstruation
-rrhea	flowing diarrhea—frequent discharge of fluid matter from the bowel
-sclerosis	hardening arteriosclerosis—hardening of the arteries
-scope	instrument for viewing laryngoscope—hollow tubes used to examine or operate upon the larynx
-tomy	a cutting operation craniotomy—cutting into the skull

-trophy,
-trophic   development, growth, nourishment
hypertrophy—overgrowth

ABBRIDGED LIST OF MEDICAL ABBREVIATIONS, SYMBOLS, AND TERMS

āā	of each
AAMA	American Association of Medical Assistants
ac	before meals
ACTH	Adrenocorticotropic hormone
ad	add
ADC	Aid to Dependent Children
ADH	Antidiuretic Hormone
ad lib	as desired; at pleasure
AFA	Aid For the Aged
AFB	Aid For the Blind
AFD	Aid For the Disabled
AIDS	Acquired Immune Deficiency Syndrome
AMA	American Medical Association
AP	Anteroposterior
aq	water
ASCVD	Ateriosclerotic Cardiovascular Disease
ASHD	Arteriosclerotic Heart Diseases
bid	twice a day
BMR	Basal Metabolic Rate
BP	Blood Pressure
c̄	with
Ca	Calcium
CA	Cancer
CAT or C-T Scan	Computerized Axial Tomography or Computerized Tomography
CBC	Complete Blood Count

cc	cubic centimeter
CC	Chief Complaint
CCU	Coronary Care Unit
cm	centimeter
CNS	Central Nervous System
COPD	Chronic Obstructive Pulmonary Disease
D	Dose
Dim	half
DNA	Does Not Apply
dr	dram
DX	Diagnosis
ea	each
ECG, EKG	Electrocardiogram
EEG	Electroencephalogram
EENT	Eye, Ear, Nose, and Throat
ENT	Ear, Nose, and Throat
ER	Emergency Room
et	and
FH	Family History
FSH	Follicle-Stimulating Hormone
GH	Growth Hormone
GI	Gastrointestinal
gm	gram
gr	grain
gt (gtt)	drop (drops)
GTT	Glucose Tolerance Test
GU	Genito-Urinary
gyn	gynecology
HBP	High Blood Pressure
Hct	Hematrocrit
Hgb, hb	Hemoglobin

hs	bedtime
ICU	Intensive Care Unit
IV	Intravenous
LH	Luteinizing Hormone
LLQ	Left Lower Quadrant
LPN	Licensed Practical Nurse
LTH	prolactin
LUQ	Left Upper Quadrant
mg	milligram
MI	Myocardial Infarction
ml	milliliter
mm	millimeter
neg	negative
NYD	Not Yet Diagnosed
OB/GYN	Obstetrics/Gynecology
OD	right eye
om	every morning
on	every night
OR	Operating Room
OS	left eye
OU	both eyes
oz	ounce
P	Pulse
PA	Posteroanterior
P & A	Percussion and Auscultation
PAP	Papanicolaou Smear
pc	after meals
prn	as needed
PTH	Parathyroid Hormone
qh	every hour
qid	four times a day

qt	*qu*art
RBC	*R*ed *B*lood *C*ells or *R*ed *B*lood (*C*ell) *C*ount
RLQ	*R*ight *L*ower *Q*uadrant
RUQ	*R*ight *U*pper *Q*uadrant
s̄	without
SIDS	*S*udden *I*nfant *D*eath *S*yndrome
sig	let it be labeled
sign	directions
sol	*sol*utions
stat	immediately
T3	*Tri*iodothyronine
T4	*T*hyroxine
Tb	*T*u*b*erculosis
temp	*temp*erature
tid	three times a day
TPR	*T*emperature, *P*ulse, *R*espiration
TSH	*T*hyroid-*S*timulating *H*ormone
UA	*U*rin*a*lysis
UCR	*U*sual, *C*ustomary, and *R*easonable
UGI	*U*pper *G*astro*i*ntestinal
URI	*U*pper *R*espiratory *I*nfection
UTI	*U*rinary *T*ract *I*nfection
VD	*V*eneral *D*isease
WBC	*W*hite *B*lood *C*ells or *W*hite *B*lood (*C*ell) *C*ount

HELPFUL PUBLICATIONS

Austrin, Miriam G. ***Young's Learning Medical Terminology Step by Step,*** 5h ed. St. Louis: C.V. Mosby Co., 1983

Birmingham, Jacqueline J. ***Medical Terminology: A Self-Learning Module.*** New York: McGraw-Hill Book Co., 1981.

Brady's Introduction to Medical Terminology, 2d ed. Bowie: Brady Communications Co., Inc., 1983.

Casady, Mona. *Word/Information Processing Concepts*. Cincinnati: South-Western Publishing Co., 1984.

Cassel, Don. *Wordstar Simplified for the IBM Personal Computer*. Englewood Cliffs: Prentice-Hall, Inc., 1984.

Dolecheck, Carolyn Crawford, and Danny W. Murphy. *Applied Word Processing*. Cincinnati: South-Western Publishing Co., 1983.

Dorland's Illustrated Medical Dictionary, 26h ed. Philadelphia: W.B. Saunders Co., 1981.

Dox, Ida, Gilbert M. Eisner, and Biagio Melloni. *Melloni's Illustrated Medical Dictionary*. Baltimore: Williams & Wilkins Co., 1979.

Dusseau, John, and Sheila B. Sloane. *A Word Book in Pathology and Laboratory Medicine*. Philadelphia: W.B. Saunders Co., 1984.

Forman, Robert E., Peter Roody, and Howard B. Schweitzer. *Medical Abbreviations and Acronyms*. New York: McGraw-Hill Book Co., 1976.

Gylys, Barbara A., and Mary E. Wedding. *Medical Terminology: A Systems Approach*. Philadelphia: F.A. Davis Co., 1983.

Hafer, Ann R. (ed.). *Medical and Health Sciences Word Book*, 2d ed. Boston: Houghton Mifflin Co., 1982.

Hall, June, and Ina Yenerich. *Business Administration for the Medical Assistant*. Colwell Co., 1983.

Hayden, Adaline C., and Edward T. Thompson. *Medical Science for Medical Record Personnel*. Berwyn: Physician's Record Co., 1974.

Jablonski, Stanley. *Illustrated Dictionary of Dentistry*. Philadelphia: W.B. Saunders Co., 1982.

Mosby's Medical Speller. St. Louis: C.V. Mosby Co., 1983.

Sellars, Dot. *Computerizing Your Medical Office: A Guide for Physicians and Their Staffs*. Oradell: Medical Economics Books, 1983.

Sloane, Sheila B. *The Medical Word Book*. Philadelphia: W.B. Saunders Co., 1982.

Stedman's Medical Dictionary, 24h ed. Baltimore: Williams & Wilkins Co., 1981.

Thomas, Clayton L. (ed.). *Taber's Cyclopedic Medical Dictionary*, 14h ed. Philadelphia: F.A. Davis Co., 1981.

Webster's Medical Speller. Springfield: Merriam-Webster, Inc., 1975.

Willeford, George, Jr. *Medical Word Finder*, 3d ed. Englewood Cliffs: Prentice-Hall, Inc., 1983.

PROFESSIONAL ORGANIZATIONS AND INFORMATION

American Association for Medical Transcription, P.O. Box 6187, Modesto, CA 95355 (Branches throughout the United States and Canada. Write for the address of the branch nearest you.)

American Association of Medical Assistants, 20 N. Wacker Dr., Suite 1575, Chicago, IL 60606

American Medical Records Association, 875 N. Michigan Avenue, Suite 1850, Chicago, IL 60611

Index

Numbers refer to paragraph numbers unless otherwise indicated.

A

AAMA Code of Ethics, 2.2
Abbreviations:
   initials and, in alphabetic indexing, 7.10
   for states, districts, territories, 6.29
Accession book, 7.25
   illustration, p. 122
Accounting:
   computerized, 14.1-14-11
   procedures for, 11.1-11.8
Account management, 14.1
Active voice, 15.4
Address placement on envelopes,
   illustration, p. 102
Adjectives, 15.3
   compound, 19.1
Admitting history, 5.13
Advance, how to, 1.16
Adverbs, 15.5
Aged-accounts receivables reports, 14.9
   illustration, p. 209
Age identifiers, 16.4
Agencies, employment, 1.7
Aggressiveness, 3.12
Aging accounts, 12.4
Air transportation, 9.1
Allowed/aloud, 15.8
All ready/already, 15.8
All right/alright, 15.8
Alphabetic card file, 7.26
   illustration, p. 123
Alphabetic filing guides and tabs, 7.22
   illustration, p. 118

Alphabetic filing procedures, 7.24
Alphabetic indexing, pp. 108-121
   abbreviations, 7.10
   businesses, names of, 7.8
   coined words, 7.20
   compound names, 7.19
   cross-referencing, 7.23
   filing guides and tabs, 7.22
   filing procedures, 7.24
   foreign language prefixes, 7.14
   government names, 7.21
   identical names, 7.15
   indexing units, order of, 7.7
   initials, 7.10
   institutions, 7.17
   married women, 7.13
   numerals in business names, 7.16
   organizations, 7.17
   possessives, 7.11
   separated single words, 7.18
   small words, 7.9
   symbols, 7.9
   titles, 7.12
American Association of Medical
   Assistants (AAMA), 2.2
American Medical Association (AMA), 2.1-2.3
   Judicial Council, 2.1
   Principles of Medical Ethics, 2.2
   Universal Health Claim form, 10.13
     illustration, p. 159
Among/between, 15.8
Ampersand, 17.1

Answering service, 4.17
Any one/anyone, 15.8
Apostrophe, 17.2
Application forms, 1.9
   illustration, pp. 7-8
Application letter, 1.12
   illustration, p. 13
Appointment book, pp. 131-140
   description of, 8.1
   for a group practice, illustration, p. 133
   for a single practice, illustration, p. 132
Appointment card for follow-up, illustration, p. 139
Appointments, 4.2
   cancelling, 8.9
   daily list of, 8.7
      illustration, p. 137
   follow-up, 8.13
   missed, 8.10
   nonpatient, 8.11
   patient referral, 4.10
   patients without, 8.12
   recording, 8.4
   record of lengthy, illustration, p. 134
   record of routine, illustration, p. 134
   reminder of missed, illustration, p. 138
   reminding patients of, 4.11
   rescheduling, 8.8
   routine, 8.2
Assertiveness, 3.12
Assigning payment to the physician, 10.9
Asterisk, 17.3
Attention line, 6.17
Audit trails, 10.14
Authority to operate form, 5.24
   illustration, p. 78
Authorization for records release, 5.23
Authorization to release information, illustration, p. 78
Automated files, 7.5
Automated office, 1.15
Automatic cross-posting, 14.8

B

Bad/badly, 15.8
Beside/besides, 15.8
Bibliographies, sexual identifiers in, 16.3
Billing, pp. 177-181
   external, 12.1
   internal, 12.2
Billing charges and insurance, calls about, 4.2
Billing periods, 12.3
Billings and collections reports, computerized, 14.11
Billing statement, computerized, 14.6
   illustration, p. 208
Bioethics, 2.3
Blind copy notation, 6.23
Block letter style, 6.11
   illustration, p. 85
Blood tests, 5.9
   reporting form for, illustration, p. 68
Blue Cross/Blue Shield, 10.2
Body of letter, 6.19
   capitalization in, 18.2
Brace/brackets, 17.4
Businesses, names of:
   in alphabetic indexing, 7.8
   capitalization of, 18.3
Business letter. *See* letter, business

C

Call-back message, illustration, p. 57
Call-in emergencies, 3.20
Calls:
   collect, 4.12
   conference, 4.14
   long distance, 4.12
   outside local, 4.9
   person-to-person, 4.12
   screening, 4.2
   station-to-station, 4.12
Cancelling appointments, 8.9
Capital/capitol, 15.8

Capitalization, pp. 252-259
   basics of, 18.1
   in business letters, 18.2
   of businesses, 18.3
   educational titles, 18.4
   government, 18.5
   with hyphenation, 18.6
   of institutions, 18.3
   nouns including letters or numbers, 18.7
   persons, 18.8
   personal and professional titles, 18.9
   places, things, and ideas, 18.10
   publications, 18.11
   time, 18.12
Carbon copy notation, 6.23
Case history, 5.3
   illustration, p. 64
Case of pronouns, 15.2
Certificates, 1.10
Certification of illness or health by physician, 5.21
   illustration, p. 76
CHAMPUS, 10.7
CHAMPVA, 10.7
Character traits, important medical office employee, 3.6-3.13
Check register, computerized, 14.7
   illustration, p. 208
Chronological or integrated record, 5.18
Civilian Health and Medical Program of the Uniformed Services (CHAMPUS), 10.7
Civilian Health and Medical Program of the Veteran's Administration (CHAMPVA), 10.7
Claim form:
   general guidelines for completing, 10.12
   superbill used with insurance, illustration, p. 156
Claim register, 10.14
   illustration, p. 163
Classes of mail, 6.36
Closed patient files, 7.2
Coined words in alphabetic indexing, 7.20

Collect calls, 4.12
Collecting from patients, pp. 181-189
Collection letter series, 12.5
   illustration, pp. 184-185
Collections reports, computerized, 14.11
Collections when insurance is involved, 12.6
Colon, 17.5
Color-coded ledger card showing overdue balance, illustration, p. 182
Color codes, illustration, p. 128
Color coding:
   for different physicians, 7.39
   patient names, 7.37
   patient numbers, 7.38
Colored folder tabs with open-shelf filing cabinets, 7.36
Comma, 17.6
Common nouns, 15.1
Communications, verbal and nonverbal, p. 35
Complimentary close, 6.20
   capitalization of, 18.2
Composing letters for the doctor's signature, 6.27
Compound adjectives, 19.1
Compound names in alphabetic indexing, 7.19
Compound nouns, 15.1, 19.3
   sexual identifiers in, 16.1
Compound pronouns, 15.2
Computer equipment, configuring, 14.19
Computer information screen, illustration, p. 203
Computerized:
   accounting, pp. 202-210
   billing statement, 14.6
      illustration, p. 208
   check and cash register, 14.7
      illustration, p. 208
   daily log, 14.4
      illustration, p. 205
   data base management, 14.12
   insurance forms, 14.5

illustration, p. 207
labels, 14.14
patient ledger, 14.3
   illustration, p. 205
records, 7.42
statement, 12.2
   illustration, p. 180
superbill, 14.2
   illustration, p. 204
Computers:
   confidentiality and, pp. 215-217
   electronic communication by, 14.25
   memory capacity of, 14.18
   types of, 14.17
Computer security, AMA position on, 14.26
Conference calls, 4.14
Confidential information about the doctor, 2.10
Confidentiality, 3.7, 5.19
   computers and, pp. 215-217
   privilege of patient, 2.5
Configuring computer equipment, 14.19
Conjunctions, 15.7
Consent, patient, 2.15
Consent form, illustration, p. 30
Consideration, 3.5
Consultation report, 5.15
   illustration, p. 72
Contractions, apostrophes and, 17.2
Controlled Substances Act, 2.22
Copy notation, 6.23
Correspondence, preparing the doctor's, 6.9-6.27
Correspondence files, 7.3
   miscellaneous, 7.28
Cover letter. *See* Job inquiry letter
CPT-4 (Current Procedural Terminology, 4h ed.), 10.10, 11.1
Cross posting, automatic, 14.8
Cross-referencing, 7.23
   in alphabetic filing, 7.23
   card for, illustration, pp. 119-121
   in geographic filing, 7.33
   of subject files, 7.30

Current Procedural Terminology (CPT-4), 10.01, 11.1
Curriculum vitae. *See* resume
Cycle billing, 12.3
Cytopathology, 5.11
   report for, illustration, p. 69

D

Daily list of appointments, 8.7
   illustration, p. 137
Daily log, 11.3
   computerized, 14.4
     illustration, p. 205
   superbill and, illustration, p. 172
Dash, 17.7
Data base management, pp. 210-212
   computerized, 14.12
Data base system, 13.3
Data processing, 1.15
Date incoming mail, 6.4
Dateline in business letters, 6.14
   capitalization of, 18.2
   placement of, table, p. 87
Delivering mail, 6.7
Delivering messages, 4.8
Dependability, 3.8
Depositing the day's receipts, 11.8
Depositions, 2.18
Deposit slip, illustration, p. 175
Diagnosis-related groups, 10.10
Dictionary of Occupational Titles (DOT), 16.1
Directory assistance, 4.15
Disability certificate, 5.22
   illustration, p. 78
Discharge summary, 5.14
   illustration, p. 71
Diskettes, floppy, 14.20
Disks, hard, 14.20
Display Write, 13.5
Distributing with word processing, 13.7
Dispensing drugs, 2.22
District abbreviations, 6.29
Doctor's notes, 5.5
   illustration, p. 65

Double booking, 8.5
DRGs, 10.01
Drugs:
    dispensing, 2.22
    prescribing, 2.23
Drug schedules, 2.24
Duplicating with word processors, 13.6

E

Ear, nose, and throat (ENT), 1.6
Educational terms, capitalization of, 18.4
Electrocardiogram, 5.8
    report for, illustration, p. 67
Electronic appointment scheduling, 14.16
Electronic communication, 14.25
Electronic typewriter, 13.3
Emergencies, 3.2
    appointments for, 8.3
    call-in, 3.20
    handling, 3.19-3.20
    walk-in, 3.19
Emergency hospital treatment, 8.17
Emergency medical care, arranging for, 3.20
Emergency telephone calls, 3.20
Employee skills, most requested, p. 3
Employment agencies, 1.7
Employment opportunities in medical offices, 1.1-1.5
    finding, 1.7-1.14
    where to look for, 1.7
Employment tests, 1.10
Enclosure notation, 6.22
End-of-day financial activities, 11.7
Envelope address placement, illustration, p. 102
Envelope notations, 6.33
Envelopes, preparation of, for outgoing mail, 6.28
Ethics, medical, 2.1
Every one/everyone, 15.8
Exception to physician/patient privilege, 2.6

Exclamation mark, 17.9
Expense account forms, 9.6
External billing, 12.1

F

Facsimile machine, 13.3
Family practice, 1.6
Family relationship words, 19.7
Farther/further, 15.8
Fewer/less, 15.8
File copies, 6.24
File guides and tabs:
    alphabetic, 7.22
    geographic, 7.34
    numeric, 7.27
        illustration, p. 123
    subject, 7.31
Files, types of, pp. 105-108
    automated, 7.5
    geographic, pp. 126-127
    inactive and closed patient, 7.2
    microfiche and microfilm, 7.6
    miscellaneous correspondence, 7.3
    patient, 7.1
    research, 7.4
    subject, pp. 124-127
    telephone, 4.16
Filing cabinets, open-shelf, with colored folder tabs, 7.36
Filing systems, color in medical, pp. 127-129
Financial records, guidelines for completing, 11.4
Fixed dateline, 6.14
Flexibility, 3.10
Floating dateline, 6.14
Floppy diskettes, 14.20
Flow of written communications in the traditional medical office, p. 192
Folding business letters, 6.34
    illustration, p. 103
Follow-up appointments:
    arranging, 8.13
    pre-printed reminder cards for, illustrations, pp. 139-140

in several months, 8.14
Foreign language prefixes in alphabetic indexing, 7.14
Foreign travel, 9.8
Foreword/forward, 15.8
Formally/formerly, 15.8
Form letters, 13.4
Forms:
   patient-completed, 5.1-5.2
   physician-completed, 5.3-5.5
Forth/fourth, 15.8
Fractions, hyphenation of, 19.4
Friendliness, 3.4

G

General practice, 1.6
Generic pronouns, sexual identifiers in, 16.2
Geographic filing systems, pp. 126-127
   cross-referencing of, 7.33
   filing guides and tabs in, 7.34
   illustration, p. 127
   procedures for, 7.35
Good Samaritan laws, 2.21
Good/well, 15.8
Government names:
   in alphabetic indexing, 7.21
   capitalization of, 18.5
Graphics software, 14.23
Greeting:
   new patients, 3.15
   patients and other visitors, 3.14-3.16
   returning patients, 3.14
   visitors other than patients, 3.16
Gross negligence, 2.11
Ground transportation, 9.2
Group health insurance, 10.1

H

Hard disks, 14.20
Hardware, pp. 212-213
Headings, capitalization of, in business letters, 18.2
Health, certification of, 5.21

Health care coverage, types of, pp. 148-152
   Blue Cross/Blue Shield, 10.2
   CHAMPUS/CHAMPVA, 10.7
   health insurance, 10.1
   Health Maintenance Organizations, 10.3
   Medicaid, 10.6
   Medicare, 10.5
   Preferred Provider Organization, 10.4
   Workers' Compensation, 10.8
Health insurance, pp. 148-165
Health Maintenance Organizations (HMOs), 10.3
Helping verbs, 15.4
History:
   admitting, 5.13
   case, 5.3
Holding, 4.7
Honesty, 3.6
Horizontal measures in typing, p. 83
Hospital:
   employment opportunities in, 1.3
   non-surgical treatment in the, 8.15
   permission for, to release information, illustration, p. 24
   scheduling patients for the, pp. 140-141
   surgery in the, 8.16
Hospital reports, 5.13-5.15
Hospital treatment, emergency, 8.17
Hospital visits, recording charges for, 11.5
Hotel reservations, 9.3
Human relations skills, p. 3
   consideration, 3.5
   friendliness, 3.4
   patience, 3.1
   poise, 3.2
   sensitivity, 3.3
Hyphen, 17.10
Hyphenated names in signature lines, 6.20
Hyphenation, pp. 260-263
   capitalization with, 18.6
   compound adjectives, 19.2

compound nouns, 19.3
family relationships, 19.7
fractions, 19.4
other uses of, 19.8
ranges, 19.5
suspended, 19.6
word division, 19.1

I

ICDA, 10.10
Ideas, capitalization of, 18.10
Identical names in alphabetic indexing, 7.15
Identification ledger, patient, 7.25
Illness:
    calls concerning, 4.2
    certification of, 5.21
Inactive patient files, 7.2
Incoming mail, 6.1-6.8
    attach related files to, 6.6
    date the, 6.4
    delivering, 6.7
    logging, 6.8
    opening, 6.1
    reviewing, 6.2
    save return address, 6.3
    sorting, 6.5
Indefinite pronouns, 15.2
Indexing, alphabetic, pp. 108-121
Indexing units, order of, 7.7
Individual health insurance, 10.1
Information:
    confidential, about the doctor, 2.10
    personal, about patients, 2.8
    releasing, inadvertently, 2.9
Initials in alphabetic indexing, 7.10
Inquiries, patient, 2.7
Inside address, 6.16
    capitalization of, 18.2
Institutions:
    in alphabetic indexing, 7.17
    capitalization of, 18.3
Insurance:
    calls about billing charges and, 4.2
    health, 10.1

    letter to patient asking for information about, illustration, p. 186
    malpractice or professional liability, 2.16
Insurance claim form:
    filing, pp. 152-165
    guidelines for completing, 10.12
    superbill with, illustration, p. 156
Insurance coding system, 10.10
Insurance company:
    letter seeking information from, illustration, p. 187
    permission to release information to, illustration, p. 23
Insurance forms, computerized, 14.5
    illustration, p. 207
Insurance rejection, letter to patient regarding, illustration, p. 187
Integrated applications programs, 13.3
Integrated record, chronological or, 5.18
Internal billing, 12.2
Internal medicine, 1.6
International Classification of Diseases, Adapted, 10.10
Interoffice memorandum, 6.26
    illustration, p. 97
Interview, 1.13
Introduction of patient, 5.20
Irregular verbs, regular and, 15.4
Itinerary, preparing an, 9.5
    illustration, p. 146
Italics, 17.16

J

Job inquiry letter, 1.8
    illustration, p. 5
Job opening ad, illustration, p. 12
Job Title Revisions to Eliminate Sex- and Age-Referent Language from the Dictionary of Occupational Titles, 16.1
Job vacancies not yet advertised, 1.7

K

Knew/new, 15.8

L

Labels, computerized, 14.14
Laboratory reports, 5.6-5.12
Laboratory requests, 5.6
  illustration, p. 66
Last/latest, 15.8
Later/latter, 15.8
Law:
  ethics and the, 2.1
  Good Samaritan, 2.21
  medical, 2.1
Lawsuits, malpractice, 21.7
  settlement of, 2.19
Leased/least, 15.8
Ledger card, 7.1, 11.2
  color-coded for overdue balance,
    illustration, p. 182
  illustration, p. 169
  as statement, 12.2
  superbill, daily log, and, illustration,
    p. 172
Lengthy appointment, recording,
  illustration, p. 134
Letter, business, 6.9-6.27
  additional pages, 6.25
  attention line, 6.17
  body, 6.19
  capitalization, 18.2
  company name, 6.20
  complimentary close, 6.20
  composing, for the doctor's signature,
    6.27
  copy notation, 6.23
  dateline, 6.14
  enclosure notation, 6.22
  file copies, 6.24
  folding, 6.34
    illustration, p. 103
  inside address, 6.16
  mailing notations, 6.15
  margins, 6.10
  medical office letterhead, 6.9
  punctuation styles:
    mixed, 6.13
    open, 6.13
  reference initials, 6.21
  salutation, 6.16
  signature lines, 6.20
  styles:
    block, 6.11
    modified block with block
      paragraphs, 6.11
    modified block with indented
      paragraphs, 6.11
  subject line, 6.17
Letter, job inquiry, *See* Job inquiry
  letter
Letter, personal, 6.12
Letterhead, 6.9
Letter margins, 6.10
  table, p. 83
Letter styles, 6.11
Liability, rule of personal, 2.13
Liable/libel, 15.8
Licensure, 2.4
Local calls, outside, 4.9
Long distance calls, 4.12
  returning, 4.13
Loose/lose, 15.8
Lotus 1 2 3, 13.3
Lotus Symphony, 13.3, 13.5
Loyalty, 3.11

M

Mail, classes of, 6.36
Mail, incoming, 6.1-6.8
  attach related files to, 6.6
  date, 6.4
  deliver, 6.7
  open, 6.1
  review, 6.2
  save the return address, 6.3
  sort, 6.5
Mail, outgoing, 6.28-6.37

Mailing address, 6.31
Mailing notations, 6.15
Mailing services, special, 6.37
Mail logs, 6.8
  illustration, p. 81
Mail merge, 13.3
Mainframe computers, 14.17
Major medical insurance, 10.1
Malpractice claims, 2.11
  preventing, 2.14
Malpractice insurance, 2.16
Malpractice lawsuits, 2.17
  settlement of, 2.19
Malpractice trials, medical, 2.20
Margins and spacing, 5.25
Married women in alphabetic indexing, 7.13
May be/maybe, 15.8
Medicaid, 10.6
  letter to patient regarding, illustration, p. 186
Medical care, arranging for emergency, 3.20
Medical centers, 1.2
Medical conditions, calls concerning, 4.2
Medical correspondence, 6.1-6.37
Medical ethics, 2.1
Medical field, finding employment in the, 1.7-1.14
Medical filing systems, color in, pp. 127-129
Medical law, 2.1
Medical messages:
  illustration, p. 53
  taking, 4.4
Medical office employee, important character traits for, 3.6-3.13
Medical offices:
  employment opportunities, in, 1.1-1.5
  traditional, 1.1
Medical records, 7.1
  problem-oriented, 5.16
  procedures, 5.16-5.19
  source-oriented, 5.17

Medical reports, procedure for typing, 5.25-5.26
Medicare, 10.5
Memorandum, interoffice, 6.26
  illustration, p. 97
Memory capacity, 14.18
Messages:
  delivering, 4.8
  general, 4.3
  medical, 4.4
Metered mail, 6.35
Microcomputers, 14.17
Microfiche, 7.6
  illustration, p. 108
Microfilm, 7.6
  illustration, p. 108
Microsoft Word, 13.5
Minicomputers, 14.17
Miscellaneous correspondence files, 7.3, 7.28
Missed appointment reminders, 8.10
  illustration, p. 138
Mixed punctuation, 6.13
Modified block letter style:
  with block paragraphs, 6.11
    illustration, p. 85
  with indented paragraphs, 6.11
    illustration, p. 86
Monthly billing, 12.3

N

Names:
  of businesses in alphabetic indexing, 7.8
  color coding patient, 7.37
  hyphenated, in signature lines, 6.20
Negligence, 2.11
Networking, 13.3
Neurology, 1.6
Nine-digit expanded ZIP Code, 6.32
Nominative case, 15.2
Nonpatient appointments, 8.11
Non-surgical treatment in the hospital, 8.15

Nonverbal communications, p. 35
Nouns, 15.1
  compound, 19.3
    sexual identifiers in, 16.1
  including letters and numbers, capitalization of, 18.7
Number, color coding patient, 7.38
Numerals in alphabetic indexing, 7.16
Numeric filing, pp. 121-124
  file guides and tabs for, 7.27
    illustration, p. 123
  procedures for, 7.29
Nutrient Analysis, 13.3

O

Objective case, 15.2
Obstetrics/Gynecology (OB/GYN), 1.6
Office technology, 1.15
Office Writer, 13.5
Official Airline Guide (OAG), 9.1
Officials and titles, capitalization of, 18.5
Opening the mail, 6.1
Open punctuation, 6.13
Open-shelf filing cabinets with colored folder tabs, 7.36
Operate, authority to, 5.24
Opthalmology, 1.6
Optical scanners, 13.3
Organizations:
  in alphabetic indexing, 7.17
  professional, 1.16
Originating processes with word processing, 13.4
Orthopedics, 1.6
Outgoing mail, pp. 98-104
  classes of, 6.36
  envelope notations, 6.33
  folding business letters, 6.34
  mailing address, 6.31
  metered mail, 6.35
  nine-digit expanded ZIP Codes, 6.32
  preparation of envelopes, 6.28
  return address, 6.30
  special mailing service, 6.37
  two-letter state and provincial abbreviations, 6.29
Out guides, 7.40
Outside local calls, 4.9
Overdue balance, color-coded ledger card showing, illustration, p. 182

P

Parentheses, 17.11
Parts of speech, pp. 218-232
  adjectives, 15.3
  adverbs, 15.5
  conjunctions, 15.7
  nouns, 15.1
  prepositions, 15.6
  problem parts of speech, 15.8
  pronouns, 15.2
  verbs, 15.4
Passed/past, 15.8
Passive voice, 15.4
Pathology reports, 5.11
Patience, 3.1
Patient alphabetic card, illustration, p. 123
Patient-completed forms, 5.1-5.2
Patient confidentiality, privilege of, 2.5
Patient consent, 2.15
Patient files, 7.1
  creating, pp. 129-130
    using computerized records for, 7.42
    instructions for, 7.41
  inactive and closed, 7.2
Patient health questionnaire, 5.2
  illustration, p. 63
Patient identification ledger, 7.25
Patient information form, 5.1
  illustration, p. 61
Patient inquiries, 2.7
Patient ledger, computerized, 14.3
  illustration, p. 205
Patient names, color coding, 7.37
Patient numbers, color coding, 7.38
Patient referral form, illustration, p. 76

Patients:
   greeting, 3.14-3.16
      new, 3.15
      returning, 3.14
   introduction of, 5.20
   reminding, of appointments, 4.11
   responding to questions from, 4.5
Payments received in the mail, recording, 11.6
Pediatrics, 1.6
Pegboard accounting, pp. 166-176
Period, 17.12
Permission for hospital to release information, p. 24
Permission to release information to insurance company, illustration, p. 23
Personal business letter, 6.12
   illustration, p. 86
Personal calls, handling the doctor's, 4.6
Personal computer:
   hardware, 13.3
   software, 13.3
Personal data sheet. *See* resume.
Personal information about patients, 2.8
Personal/personnel, 15.8
Personal pronouns, 15.2
Personal titles, capitalization of, 18.9
Persons, capitalization of, 18.8
Person-to-person call, 4.12
Photocopy notation, 6.23
Physical examination form, 5.4
   illustration, p. 64
Physician:
   notation to show unavailability of, illustration, p. 135
   responsibility of, for employees, 2.12
   specialty areas of, 1.6
Physician-completed forms, 5.3-5.5
Physician/patient privilege, exception to, 2.6
Physicians' Current Procedural Terminology, 10.10
Physician's Office Computer, 14.1

Places, capitalization of, 18.10
Plurals, apostrophes and, 17.2
P.M.S. Medical Billing System, 13.3
Poise, 3.2
Possession, apostrophes and, 17.2
Possessive case, 15.2
Possessives in alphabetic indexing, 7.11
Posted or advertised positions, 1.7
Preferred Provider Organization (PPO), 10.4
Prepositions, 15.6
Preprinted follow-up reminder card, illustration, p. 140
Prescribing drugs, 2.23
Prescription refills, calls for, 4.2
Principal/principle, 15.8
Privacy, 3.3
Privilege of patient confidentiality, 2.5
Problem-oriented medical record, 5.16
   illustration, p. 74
Producing and revising word processing, 13.5
Production report analysis, 14.10
Professionalism, 3.13
Professional liability insurance. *See* malpractice insurance
Professional Liability in the 80s, 2.11
Professional organizations, 1.16
Professional titles, capitalization of, 18.9
Progress notes, 5.5
Pronouns, 15.2
   sexual identifiers in generic, 16.2
Proofreader's marks, illustration, p. 197
Proper nouns, 15.1
Provincial abbreviations, 6.29
Publications, capitalization of, 18.11
Punctuation, pp. 237-251
   ampersand, 17.1
   apostrophe, 17.2
   asterisks, 17.3
   brace/brackets, 17.4
   colon, 17.5
   comma, 17.6
   dash, 17.7

exclamation mark, 17.9
hyphen, 17.10
italics, 17.16
parentheses, 17.11
period, 17.12
question mark, 17.13
quotation mark, 17.14
semicolon, 17.15
slash, 17.8
underscore, 17.16
Punctuation styles in business letters, 6.13

Q

Question mark, 17.13
Quotation in letter, 6.19
Quotation marks, 17.14

R

Radiology reports, 5.10
   illustration, p. 69
Ranges, 19.5
Real/really, 15.8
Recall notices, 14.13
Reception area:
   maintenance of, 3.17-3.18
   setting up the, 3.17
Recording payments received in the mail, 11.6
Record procedures, medical, 5.16-5.19
Records release, authorization for, 5.23
Reference initials in letters, 6.21
Referral appointments, making patient, 4.10
Regular verbs, irregular and, 15.4
Releasing information inadvertently, 2.9
Reminder notices, 14.13
   for missed appointments, illustration p. 130
   preprinted follow-up, illustration, p. 140
Reminding patients of appointments, 4.11

Reports:
   consultation, 5.15
   hospital, 5.13-5.15
   laboratory, 5.6-5.12
      shingled, 5.12
         illustration, p. 70
   pathology, 5.11
   radiology, 5.10
Research, 14.15
Research centers, employment opportunities in, 1.4
Research files, 7.4
   illustration, p. 107
Rescheduling appointments, 8.8
Responding to patients' questions, 4.5
Responsibility, physician's, for employees, 2.12
Resume, 1.8, 1.9, 1.11
   illustration, p. 10
Return address:
   on incoming mail, 6.3
   on outgoing mail, 6.30
Returning long distance calls, 4.13
Revising word processing, 13.5
Rotary telephone number file, illustration, p. 59
Routine appointments, recording, 8.2
   illustration, p. 134
Routine reception area maintenance, 3.18
Rule of personal liability, 2.13

S

Salutation, 6.16
   capitalization of, 18.2
Screening calls, 4.2
Scheduling, pp. 131-141
   for the hospital and other medical facilities, pp. 140-141
   special, 8.6
   for therapy, X-ray, tests, and other medical services, 8.18
Self-confidence, 3.9
Semicolon, 17.15

Sensitivity, 3.3
Separated single words in alphabetic indexing, 7.18
Settlement of a malpractice lawsuit, 2.19
Sexual identifiers:
  in bibliographies, 16.3
  in compound nouns, 16.1
  in generic pronouns, 16.2
Shingled lab reports, 5.12
  illustration, p. 70
Signature line, 6.20
Skills, most requested employee, p. 3
Slash, 17.8
Small words in alphabetic indexing, 7.9
Software, pp. 213-215
  checklist for purchase of, 14.22
  graphics, 14.23
  selection of, 14.21
  word processing, 14.24
Some/sum, 15.8
some time/sometime/sometimes, 15.8
Sorting mail, 6.5
Source-oriented medical record, 5.17
Spacing, margins and, 5.25
Speciality areas of physicians, 1.6
Special mailing services, 6.37
Special scheduling, 8.6
Spreadsheet, 13.3
Stand-alone (dedicated) word processors, 13.1
Standardized medical letters, 13.4
  illustration, p. 196
State abbreviations, 6.29
  table, pp. 98-99
Statement form, 12.2
  illustrations, pp. 179-180
Station-to-station call, 4.12
Storing with word processing, 13.8
Subject, agreement of verb and, 15.4
Subject filing, pp. 124-127
  cross-referencing of, 7.30
  filing guides and tabs for, 7.31
  illustration of, p. 125
  procedures for, 7.32

Subject line, 6.18
Superbill, 11.1
  with claim form, illustration, p. 156
  computerized, 14.2
    illustration, p. 204
  with CPT and ICDA codes,
    illustration, p. 155
  daily log and, illustration, p. 172
  with hospital charges, illustration, p. 174
  illustration, p. 167
  as insurance claim documentation, 10.11
  ledger card and, illustration, p. 172
  as statement, 12.2
Sure/surely, 15.8
Surgery, 1.6
  in the hospital, 8.16
Suspended hyphenation, 19.6
Symbols in alphabetic indexing, 7.9

T

Tables, 5.26
Tabs, filing guides and:
  alphabetic, 7.22
  numeric, 7.27
    illustration, p. 123
  open-shelf filing cabinets with colored, 7.36
Technology, office, 1.15
Telecommunications software, 13.3
Telephone, answering the, 4.1-4.8
Telephone calls:
  collect, 4.12
  conference, 4.14
  emergency, 3.20
  long distance, 4.12
  outside local, 4.9
  person-to-person, 4.12
  screening, 4.2
  station-to-station, 4.12
Telephone message form, illustration, p. 51
Telephone number file, 4.16
  illustration of rotary, p. 59

Tense of verbs, 15.4
  table, p. 226
Territory abbreviations, 6.29
  table, pp. 98-99
Test results, calls for, 4.2
Tests:
  blood, 5.9
  employment, 1.10
  scheduling for, 8.18
Than/then, 15.8
Thank-you letter to interviewer, 1.14
  illustration, p. 15
Their/there, 15.8
Therapy, scheduling for, 8.18
Tickler file, 10.14
  illustration, p. 164
Time, capitalization of, 18.12
Titles, personal and professional:
  in alphabetic indexing, 7.12
  capitalization of, 18.5, 18.9
To/too/two, 15.8
Traditional medical offices, 1.1
Transcription, 13.3
Travel arrangements, pp. 142-147
Traveler's checks, 9.4
Traveler's package, 9.7
Trials, medical malpractice, 2.20
Truth in lending disclosure, 12.7
  illustration, p. 189
Typing measures, horizontal and
    vertical, p. 83
Typing medical reports, procedure for,
    5.25-5.26

U

Underscore, 17.16
Unethical, 2.1
Universal Health Insurance Claim
    Form, 10.13
  illustration, p. 159
Urinalysis report, 5.7
  illustration, p. 66
Urine test. *See* Urinalysis report
Urology, 1.6

V

Variable information for standardized
    letter, illustration, p. 196
Verb, agreement of subject and, 15.4
Verbal communications, p. 35
Verb tense, 15.4
  table, p. 226
Vertical measures in typing, p. 83
Visitors, greeting, 3.16
Voice of verbs, 15.4

W

Walk-in emergencies, 3.19
Walk-in patients, 8.12
Weak/week, 15.8
Weather/whether, 15.8
Word division, 19.1
Word processing, 1.15
  defined, 13.1
  future of, 13.9
  how it works, 13.3
  stages of:
    distributing, 13.7
    duplicating, 13.6
    originating, 13.4
    producing and revising, 13.5
    storing, 13.8
  why it is used, 13.2
Word processing menus, 13.3
Word processing software, 14.24
Wordstar, 13.5
Workers' Compensation, 10.8
  claim form for, illustration, p. 153
  letter to employer regarding,
    illustration, p. 188

XYZ

X-rays, 5.10
  scheduling for, 8.18
ZIP Code, nine-digit, 6.32

By matching the guides at the edge of this page with the marks opposite them along the edge of the book, you can quickly turn to the unit containing the material you want.

1. OVERVIEW
2. MEDICAL ETHICS AND MEDICAL LAW
3. INTERPERSONAL SKILLS
4. TELEPHONE COMMUNICATION
5. MEDICAL FORMS AND MEDICAL REPORTS
6. MEDICAL CORRESPONDENCE
7. MEDICAL OFFICE FILES
8. SCHEDULING
9. TRAVEL ARRANGEMENTS
10. HEALTH INSURANCE CLAIMS
11. ACCOUNTING PROCEDURES IN THE MEDICAL OFFICE
12. MEDICAL BILLING AND COLLECTIONS
13. WORD PROCESSING IN THE MEDICAL OFFICE
14. THE COMPUTER AND THE MEDICAL OFFICE
15. PARTS OF SPEECH
16. ELIMINATING BIAS IN WRITING
17. PUNCTUATION
18. CAPITALIZATION
19. HYPHENATION

APPENDIX